BEDSIDE MANNER

HOW TO GAIN YOUR PATIENTS' RESPECT, LOVE & LOYALTY

DR. ROBERT M. FLEISHER

uphill books

A special thanks to the many patients who, over the years, have taught me what I now pass on to future generations of healthcare providers. With deep gratitude I dedicate this book to the many doctors, nurses, assistants and associated healthcare providers for sharing their stories, philosophies and techniques to help develop this book. And finally, I want to thank my wonderful family and dear friends who have helped me through life's journey and have had to put up with my constant lecturing.

CONTENTS

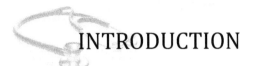

INTRODUCTION

Dr. Jones goes to the nursing home for his monthly
rounds. He sees Joe and asks him, "Joe, how much
is three times three?" Joe replies, "Fifty-nine." He
goes over to Tom and asks him, "How much is three
times three?" Tom replies, "Wednesday." Finally, he
goes over to John and asks him, "How much is three
times three?" "Nine," replies John. "That's right. Now
how did you come to that answer?" "It was easy;
I just subtracted fifty-nine from Wednesday."

Bedside manner is a skill set that requires understanding and addressing the psychology of patients who present with needs, hopes, and fears. Doctors with great bedside manner have loyal patients who will want to stay under their care, refer new patients, and almost never bring suit even when things don't go well. Being a great doctor requires a constant effort to develop and maintain interpersonal skills. It is just too easy to get preoccupied with the art and science of your profession and forget to take the time to deal with the human being attached to the chart.

Being considerate and having a sense of humor are two of the many components of bedside manner. To be a truly great doctor you must address all of the elements, many of which are not so obvious. Exploring everything from communication skills to character issues provides many ways to improve the doctor patient relationship, and that is what bedside manner is all about.

A practitioner devoid of any semblance of bedside manner, who is more concerned with productivity than patient care, received this actual letter from a clergyman who was unhappy with his experience. You never want to get a letter like this.

> *Dear "Friends"*
>
> *Please find the enclosed check ($180) for my visit to your office.*
>
> *Unfortunately, I find it difficult to pay such a large amount of money for one of the most impersonal, unprofessional and unpleasant experiences I have had in many years.*
>
> *May I suggest an attempt to reduce a factory like experience as well as your excessive disclaimers for insurance monies and make an effort to improve on friendliness. It seems I had to ask the name of the "specialist consultant" after forty minutes into the visit.*
>
> *Thanks for your time and consideration.*
>
> *Sincerely,*
>
> *Reverend xxx x xxx*

Every practitioner should strive to stand out as the best of the best. It takes a lot of effort to become the best – more than understanding the science of your chosen field. It's not only what service you deliver; it's how you deliver it.

ELEMENTS OF BEDSIDE MANNER

Patient: "Doctor, if I give up wine, women, and
smoking, will I live longer?"
Doctor: "Not really, it'll just seem longer."

B eing a great doctor and being perceived as a great doctor by your patients are two entirely different matters.

Every health-care school in the nation provides curriculum to train highly competent practitioners to serve the community. However, formal training in bedside manner, the way in which a doctor relates to the patient, is generally underdeveloped. While it may be impossible to change your personality, there is no reason basic interpersonal skills can't be learned as they relate to managing patients.

The *Seven Cs of a Great Doctor:*

1. Competency
2. Compassion
3. Communication
4. Confidence
5. Character
6. Class
7. Comedy

Ironically, competence is the only trait of a great doctor not required for great bedside manner. As patients have almost no way of determining the medical proficiency of doctors, they usually assume their doctors are knowledgeable and competent. When patients heal, that becomes validation of competency. When they don't get better, most patients still assume there are medical reasons beyond the control of their doctor. It is, therefore, the remaining six characteristics that patients use to judge their doctors.

The *Six Cs of Great Bedside Manner:*

1. Compassion
2. Communication
3. Confidence
4. Character
5. Class
6. Comedy

It is the *Six Cs of Bedside Manner* that make patients love and cherish certain doctors. These are the qualities that constitute great bedside manner.

Compassion – The ability to show you truly care about the plight of the patient.

Communication – The ability of a doctor to make the time spent with the patient meaningful. Communication is a two-way street requiring the ability to listen as well as the ability to explain. When the doctor doesn't understand the patient's problems and the patient doesn't understand the course of treatment, care is jeopardized and the opportunity to build patient loyalty is lost.

Confidence – The ability to convey to the patient that you are competent and have all the ability to solve their problems.

Confidence is very much a communicative skill and goes hand in hand with how you communicate.

Character – Character is best defined as moral and ethical values. Character goes beyond the Hippocratic Oath. It is who you are as a person in society and it includes the values you learned from your parents and teachers.

Class – or conduct is actually the way a professional looks, acts and handles him- or herself in general and more specifically when interacting with patients.

Comedy – The ability of a doctor to make patients smile or laugh in a setting that doesn't engender much humor. Make your patients laugh and they will love you.

When patients visit the doctor, they are often scared, nervous or worried. Apprehension and fear can manifest in many ways. The patient might be verbal, quiet and withdrawn, belligerent, nervous, anxious, or outright hysterical. An amalgamation of these behaviors is common. All of these behaviors can be modified by any one of the *Six Cs of Great Bedside Manner*. Used in combination, you can make most any patient feel more comfortable.

By learning and utilizing the methods in this book, you will improve the way in which you relate to your patients and develop a great bedside manner. These skills will enable you to have enhanced medical outcomes, grow your practice, protect yourself from lawsuits, and gain your patients' respect, love, and loyalty. So let's take a look at each of the *Six Cs* in more detail.

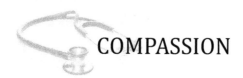

COMPASSION

After a thorough examination the doctor tells his elderly patient, "I have good news and bad news. The bad news is that you have cancer." The patient, distraught, asks, "What's the good news?" "The good news is that you also have Alzheimer's and pretty soon you'll forget you have cancer."

Compassion is the humane quality of understanding the suffering of others and wanting to do something about it. It isn't only showing concern for a major loss like the death of a loved one, for example. You can also show compassion for the patient whose financial problems force them to choose a less than ideal treatment. Compassion is being able to put yourself in another person's place. Feel what they feel.

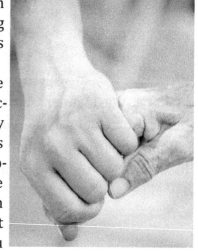

It would be nice if compassion were a universal trait that needed no instruction, but not everyone seems innately capable of understanding the problems of others, especially when those problems represent an inconvenience or are not clearly expressed. Even if you run behind schedule and want the patient to decide upon a treatment plan, or you want them to stop asking the same questions over and over, you must remain compassionate. Some patients can't express their feelings or needs and the practitioner must learn how to recognize, in a caring manner, what the patient requires.

Some practitioners have difficulty showing emotion, even when they feel it. There are others who start out empathetic then become burned out by constant exposure to sad events. It's difficult for some practitioners to understand the possibility of losing compassion, the result of burnout, but it's true. It is important to recognize the possibility, because stress and emotional detachment can cross over into relationships with family and friends. As a result, not only will your patients think you are detached, but so will your loved ones.

Whether or not you innately possess compassion, the day-to-day trials and tribulations of life can sometimes force you to become complacent and neglect the emotional needs of your patients. Fortunately, there are some simple rules that will allow you to fake it. After faking it long enough, it may actually become genuine—even if you have an inherent lack of compassion.

You treat a disease, you win, you lose. You treat a person, I guarantee you, you'll win,
no matter what the outcome.
We need to start treating the patient
as well as the disease.
—Hunter "Patch" Adams

Loss is the driving force behind the need for compassion. In health care, there are five areas of loss that require you to express compassion: loss of money (financial concerns), failing procedures, loss of function, loss of comfort, and loss of life. There are different ways to express compassion with each type of loss, but the common goal is to show you care.

LOSS OF MONEY

While fiscal matters shouldn't be part of health-care delivery, they do affect every patient. As medical practitioners we don't like to address fiscal issues, but their effect on the way doctors are perceived by patients cannot be ignored. It is difficult for a patient to respect the doctor they perceive as more concerned with money than their well-being. Fiscal policies impact how patients perceive your compassion when those policies determine the difference between obtaining proper care and being refused treatment.

A disgruntled patient: "I just couldn't go back to Dr. Smith. When I told him I couldn't afford the treatment he suggested, he told me to call him when I could find a way to make it happen. He never offered any alternatives and I felt abandoned."

Many medical doctors participate in so many insurance plans that they and their patients have no interest in discussing fees. If all treatments are fully covered, then there is no need to discuss fees. However, don't be surprised or disappointed when patients complain and refuse to pay your bill because they thought your services were covered, and they're not.

If your service requires substantial uncovered fees or large co-payments, you should make sure the patients understand their responsibility. Some doctors find it difficult to discuss money. Many practice management gurus actually don't want the doctors to discuss money with the patients. Remember, these are the same experts who show you how to make a lot of money by herding patients like cattle. They want you to limit your time to treatment planning and treatment, while they would have auxiliary staff present the financials.

You shouldn't be expected to take the money, set up payment plans, and make the next appointment; however, discussing fees, rather than delegating this task to a staff member, helps you bond with your patient. It shows that you have compassion for financial concerns.

Patients receiving treatment not covered by insurance don't like being herded into the financial arrangement office. It is very impersonal and will cause many to seek treatment from another practitioner. Those who are bullied into accepting treatment they can't afford will often become noncompliant patients who never follow through, or they will end up in collection, resulting in you performing treatment for which you never get paid.

To avoid the discontent that results in patients leaving your practice and slandering you due to financial misunderstandings, you should discuss fees and make sure the patient is aware that they are responsible for any uncovered treatment. Fiscal responsibility shouldn't be in the small print after ten pages of material your office staff asks them to read and sign. Be upfront about fees, insurance coverage, and expectations of getting paid for services rendered.

If you discuss fees compassionately, patients will see you are sensitive to their financial concerns as well as their medical problems.

After I quote a fee, I always mention that, "Root canal therapy is expensive, but it's best to try to save your tooth if you can afford it." This lets the patient know I understand potential financial concerns. It helps them discuss the issue without embarrassment.

If I quote a fee, and before I have a chance to mention how expensive it is, the patient makes a face that looks like they were just told they have a week to live, I modify my line slightly: "I know that's an awful lot of money, and while it's best to try to keep your tooth if you can afford it, there are other, less expensive alternatives."

Showing concern for the high cost of services is an expression of compassion not usually thought about by health-care providers who often don't understand that many patients cannot afford optimal care.

Even if you treat wealthy patients, never assume that a fee isn't a potential burden unless you have known the patient for many years and can take that liberty. Fees should always be quoted, in a compassionate manner, even for patients who you expect to have full insurance coverage for a particular treatment. This shows patients you understand the expense involved and it puts a value on what they receive. If it turns out that they didn't have the coverage you and they expected, they will not be totally shocked at their financial responsibility.

FAILING PROCEDURES

When a procedure fails, your patient will still hold you in high regard if you have great bedside manner. You will be better protected from legal redress if you have a proper informed consent and you have communicated the possibility of failure before the treatment. Even with these protections, you still want to express your concern and show compassion. In my specialty, that conversation could go like this:

"I'm so sorry the root canal treatment hasn't worked out for you. We tried everything possible and, unfortunately, your case was one of the ten percent that just doesn't heal."

It is best to stop at this point and wait for the patient's reaction. If they accept your statement, you should proceed with one of the following solutions:

"I'm going to make arrangements for you to have the tooth removed."

or

"I'm going to contact your dentist and let him know that he will have to make arrangements to replace this tooth."

or

"I want you to contact your dentist so he can make arrangements for you to have this tooth removed and replaced."

If the patient exhibits any feeling of discontent you proceed:

"I'm sure you remember we discussed the chance of success when we chose to give it a try."

Notice, blame is not assigned, and you remind the patient that this was what you discussed before treatment was chosen.

Sometimes the belligerent patient will deny ever having such a discussion, at which point it is time to pull out the diagram you drew explaining the treatment, or mention that it was noted in the consent they read before deciding upon treatment.

It is difficult to express compassion for a belligerent patient, but you must continue to be apologetic and explain the situation again, if necessary.

Every practitioner knows what types of failures occur in their particular field and you must have explanations for the most common questions you can expect to hear.

"Why didn't the scar fade? It looks worse than before!"

"As I explained before we decided to try this procedure, we can't predict how anyone is going to heal. Some people heal over invisibly and others develop heavy scarring. In your case, we have more of the scarring."

"How come I have more pain after the back operation than before?"

"I'm sure you remember our conversation about how we usually get a great response to this type of surgery, while other times it just doesn't work out. When there's scarring around the nerve root, it can put pressure on the nerves in the same manner that the herniated disk did before the operation."

For every procedure you perform, you must have a complete understanding of any and all complications, so that your explanations are confident, clear, legitimate, and offer comfort. Patients don't like to hear, "I've never seen anything like this before." That is not an acceptable response to their concerns. It makes them think you are incompetent. It shows no compassion. It is poor bedside manner.

Even if you have *never seen anything like that before*, try to have a good answer to help the patient deal with their concerns. This is often the case with an emotionally disturbed, petulant, or chronic pain patient.

"But doctor, ever since you removed my bunion, I noticed that my urine is green and my hair is thinning."

Although I'm not a podiatrist, I'm fairly certain those symptoms have nothing to do with the operation. Rather than getting defensive and saying, "I never heard of anything like that before," take a deep breath and try, "I'm very concerned about those symptoms you just described, especially because they have nothing to do with removing your bunion. I want you to get in touch with your medical doctor concerning this matter. I'd be happy to discuss your case in detail, if he/she wants to speak with me."

If you're the patient's medical doctor, or if you're the specialist their medical doctor sent them to, you may say you want to get a second opinion. Remember: *Every patient wants a solution.* Don't be afraid to refer them to one of your colleagues. In this manner you offer a solution without making light of their concerns or appearing defensive, which many patients interpret as incompetence or lack of compassion. Best of all, you get them into the care of someone who may be able to offer help.

Complicated cases require a cadre of specialists whom you can rely upon.

A *pain specialist* is a must-have for every practitioner, since we all see chronic pain patients or challenging pain management cases. Attempting to treat these patients without the proper expertise will be a disservice to the patient, your staff, and yourself.

It is also important to have a *psychologist/psychiatrist* for referral, but making psychiatric referrals are difficult. Patients don't like to think their problem is in their mind. The slightest mention of a psychological cause of symptoms can make the patient defensive and harbor feelings that you are not compassionate to their needs. Quite often they will doubt your expertise and seek care from other practitioners until they find one who will offer them one treatment or another, though often useless.

When you do suspect a psychological etiology, you may attempt to ease your patient into accepting a psychiatric referral: "After trying all of the methods and techniques I have at my disposal, it may be best to consider seeing a pain specialist or neurologist."

These doctors will rule out an organic etiology and make the psychiatric referral if necessary. When the patient sees, yet, another doctor who can't help them, they may finally accept the possibility that they have a psychological problem.

Since neurologists and pain specialists treat many chronic pain patients and many undiagnosed ailments, they often utilize the same antidepressants used by psychiatrists and achieve a high level of success. And when required, they have much more experience making the psychiatric referral.

THE REFERRAL PROCESS

All too many practitioners think making referrals makes them look inadequate. That is a dangerous attitude as the patient may not receive appropriate care, and the doctor places himself in jeopardy of legal redress for performing services that didn't meet the standard of care.

Making referrals shows your concern and is perceived as being compassionate as long as you do it in the appropriate manner.

It's Not Only What you Say, but How You Say It

Referrals can be perceived in two different ways:

1. NEGATIVELY: You don't want to deal with the problem, you're incompetent in your field, or you don't care about your patients.

2. POSITIVELY: You are genuinely concerned for the well-being of your patients, placing their best interest above all else.

The distinction between caring and callous does not only lie in what you say, but how you say it.

Wrong way:
"Mrs. Smith, I've never seen anything like this before. I'm almost to the point that I don't think it's your tooth that's causing the prob-

lem. I'm just not sure what it is. Doing anymore here will be a waste of time. I want to send you to a specialist."

Right way:

"Mrs. Smith, I am so sorry to see that your pain hasn't responded to any of the treatment I've done. While I can't determine why it hasn't gotten better, you most certainly have a problem, and we have to find an answer to your problem. I want you to see a doctor who specializes in hidden sources of pain. He's very good at finding why some symptoms don't respond to the usual treatments."

A variation:

"Mrs. Smith, everything we have tried is just not working. I want you to get better, and I want you to see someone who specializes in more complicated cases like yours. I'm going to send you to a doctor who has a great deal of success in cases that don't respond to conventional treatment."

This manner of referral sets up a pathway for success with the potential for placebo effect by mentioning how the new doctor has a "great deal of success." The key is to communicate compassion while maintaining your credibility. You must always be cognizant of how you are perceived by your patients.

Sometimes doctors who show great compassion and empathy become a magnet for chronic pain patients and lonely old folks. This type of patient has finally found someone who will listen to them, and they have no intention of getting better as it would end the relationship. When you refer these types of patients (after a reasonable attempt to help them), you avoid this dependency situation. If you fail to recognize this pattern, you will enable this dysfunctional behavior and you will not have time to see many patients each day.

<u>LOSS OF FUNCTION</u>

Some health-care providers treat patients who have lost function as a regular part of their practice. One might expect that the more dramatic the loss, i.e. blindness, deafness, paralysis, the more compassion needed. However, any loss of function may be considered devastating to the individual who places great value on something others may not consider. The practitioner with great bedside manner is never complacent about exhibiting the utmost compassion for any and all losses experienced by their patients.

Upon first meeting with the patient experiencing a loss of function you should acknowledge the disability with an expression of life affirming spirit.

"I could never understand what you are going through, but I can assure you I know many people dealing with your same problem, because that's my job. I am here to help them all day, every day. I'm here to help you."

If the patient is receptive, your treatment and their recovery will go well, however if the patient is in the self-pity stage of healing, other tactics may be employed.

"There are two ways you can deal with your loss, the negative way or the positive way. If you choose the negative way, you will let this loss defeat you and you will never recover. The positive way to deal with your loss is to accept it and let it make you stronger, so strong, in fact, that you will be able to deal with everything that comes your way better than most people."

You can work on your own life affirming speech, or perhaps tell the patient about some interesting or famous person who overcame the same problem and went on to conquer the world. Patients need encouragement and the knowledge that you and your team are there for them.

When you specialize in treating severely handicapped individuals, you might forget that aside from special physical needs they have special emotional needs. Treatment without compassion is not humane. I remember an internship at the head and neck cancer center where the chief of the service had us gather around severely disfigured patients while he described them as objects of interest and treated them without dignity. To show us anatomical points of interest he made each patient experience pain and gag to the point that several interns had to leave the room. He seemed to be devoid of any emotional understanding of their plight. To him these patients mattered little in the scheme of things. This doctor had no bedside manner.

LOSS OF COMFORT

Patients are often fearful and anxious when they go to their healthcare providers. Their fears can be psychological as in neuroses or obsessions, or they may be grounded in real life issues from the fear of a painful procedure to actual mortality concerns regarding a terminal diagnosis.

The doctor with great bedside manner must deal with the fears and anxieties of their patients with extra time to allow them to voice their concerns and address them, both real and perceived. Offering comfort and confidence helps to allay the patient's fears.

If the patient needs your services, and you convey to the patient that you are going to do your best and that you are the best, it offers comfort. The patient feels they are now doing everything they can to deal with their problems.

With a terminal diagnosis, it is imperative to offer hope even when there may be none based on your medical experience. There is always the possibility of miracles and you must keep that hope alive for the patient. Consider using statements like, "Even though the survival rate is low at ten percent, there is no reason you can't be in that group, and I will do everything in my power to help you be in that group."

While you should never give false hope, there is no reason to show any negativity. Humanity dictates that you always show compassion.

For the patient who is fearful of the procedure you perform, you must explain things clearly and realistically. You should inform them, "I will do everything in my power to make this as pain free as possible." Naturally you should utilize the latest, greatest techniques to minimize pain.

You don't want to lose the patient's trust by telling them things that aren't true. If there is some pain associated with a procedure, prepare them and offer encouragement, much like the hand-holding required for an apprehensive child. You may have to offer a psychological hand-holding for the fearful adult. Use distraction techniques and have your auxiliary staff talk the patient through a difficult procedure.

When a patient is in pain, you may have to address the pain before moving forward. With acute pain, as might be encountered in the emergency room, it may take more than compassion and talking to the patient. In those situations you may need to resort to medication, sedation and even anesthesia to get the patient out of acute pain. Naturally, there are times you can't achieve that goal when you need to get medical information for the safety of the patient.

Situations that involve acute pain can frustrate the practitioner and that must be suppressed. That is the time compassion is needed the most.

LOSS OF LIFE

The loss of life is so difficult for most people to accept that it requires special scripting and study to become adept at delivering the bad news in a compassionate manner, and even then, it is never easy.

For tragic situations in medicine, you will need to have prepared responses and avoid anything that sounds detached. Never say to a patient's family, "There is nothing more that I can do." While you may know this to be the case, you simply must have a better way to say the same thing.

Quite often religion is the best excuse to offer comfort when preparing a family for the end. You don't have to be religious and you can even be an outright atheist. It is not necessary to divulge your personal beliefs to comfort people at time of need. While they may curse you along with God, at least you're in good company.

"We've done everything possible to help your mother, and now it's in God's hands."

"What does that mean?"

"It means that everything medically has been tried. Now we'll see what God wants for her."

"But I don't believe in God."

"I'm truly sorry, and I hope you find comfort in your family and friends."

"I am so sorry to have to tell you this, but while we tried everything available, your father didn't make it through the operation. Though I could never feel your pain, I, too, lost someone very dear to me and my pain was overwhelming."

While some may perceive mentioning your loss as self involved, others will appreciate that you, too, shared a loss and have some understanding of their pain.

If expressions of compassion don't come naturally to you, memorize these lines and practice saying them in the mirror. Make up your own expressions of comfort, use others', and learn each time you encounter responses from grieving families that make you feel awkward. Gradually, you will develop many offerings to help comfort those in need.

Physical manifestations of compassion like the embrace, hug, and pat on the shoulder are extremely effective nonverbal tools. The use of endearing names is another important ancillary form of expressing compassion. These techniques are detailed in the chapters, *First Names, Endearing Names, and Touch* and *Delivering Bad News.*

COMMUNICATION

A terribly overweight woman goes to the doctor to find the perfect diet. "I want you to eat regularly for two days then skip a day. Do that for two weeks and when you come back you will have lost five pounds." When she returned, she shocked the doctor by losing twenty pounds. "Why, that's amazing. Did you follow my instructions?" The woman nodded. "I did, but I thought I would drop dead by the third day." "From hunger?" asked the doctor. "No, from the skipping."

The playwright George Bernard Shaw once said, "The greatest problem with communication is the illusion that it has been accomplished." In communicating healthcare information the task is all that much more of a challenge.

As one of the pillars of bedside manner, the benefit of communication cannot be overemphasized. With proper communication of expectations and instructions your patients benefit by being more compliant and thereby achieving better outcomes. You will prevent many costly, stressful, time-consuming failures that often lead to lawsuits.

Two areas of professional practice require strong communications skills: treatment plans (including description of treatment, other options, expected outcome, and postoperative sequelae), and financial considerations.

COMMUNICATING THE TREATMENT PLAN

When a patient understands their treatment plan, they have more realistic expectations of outcome, are better able to respond to adverse consequences, and they will trust and respect you even if things go wrong.

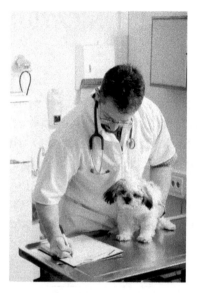

A PICTURE IS WORTH A THOUSAND WORDS

There is no better way to communicate a procedure than by employing a visual aid. You don't have to take courses in art unless your sketching skills are as bad as your handwriting. Assuming you can draw a reasonable diagram of the planned procedure, you'll be fine.

Always sit next to the patient so they can see your illustration as it comes to life. Allow them to ask questions as the need arises. At various intervals during lengthy explanations, you should ask the patient if they understand. Waiting until you are finished to answer their questions may be confusing, especially for the elderly.

Be sure to make notes alongside the drawing using key words regarding your discussion. Your notes should cover options for other forms of treatment (including the choice to doing nothing), chance for success and failure i.e. prognosis, a general explanation of the treatment procedure, postoperative considerations and cost. Make sure your explanation is understandable. Once you complete your presentation, you can give the patient a copy of the diagram.

You should be explaining things to the patient anyway, and the time it takes to make a drawing that is included in your records is well worth the effort. The diagram becomes proof that you provided a verbal informed consent. It is there to show the patient when controversy arises, such as complications, flare up or failure to achieve the expected outcome. This picture makes a great exhibit in court. While some patients don't understand no matter how hard you try, the picture shows you tried. Remember, if the jury can understand your explanation and they like your picture, they will be sympathetic to your cause.

Patients often find they can't remember or explain anything you told them when they get home. With a drawing, they have half a chance. More importantly, they appreciate your personal interest in explaining the problem and procedure in a clear and understandable manner. To provide a formal consent form based on legal advice with all sorts of disclaimers and highly complex descriptions is all right for your records, but it can't compare to an uncomplicated picture that is made personally for each patient.

Drawings are of great benefit when a patient claims they didn't understand something. In crucial instances, you will be able to calm the most aggressive of patients by producing your diagram and pointing out how you discussed the fact that the procedure may not be successful, or the fee, or the consequences of treatment.

Never rush patients when they ask questions, especially if they need to see you after you've performed a treatment and they have adverse consequences. No matter how far behind schedule you're running, rushing patients experiencing complications leads to bad will and potential lawsuits.

A Dental Specialist Says
You present differently to a CPA versus a nurse versus an engineer versus a hotel worker. What the

patient wants to know is: Do you understand the problem? Are you qualified to fix it? Can you fix it? Have you done this before? Do other people have this type of problem and will you fix it with the least amount of pain and minimal complications? It's my job to communicate the answers to these questions. Communication and trust require eye contact. I look directly into my patient's eyes when I speak with them.

––––––––––––

A major flaw in communication is to assume every patient is as knowledgeable as you are. Something as simple as a technical word you take for granted can destroy an entire explanation: "The tissue is inflamed, resulting in a productive cough."

'Tissue' is *Kleenex* to many, and 'productive' means getting the job done. While you may be smiling at the absurdity of this example, it is not at all absurd, and you will understand this when you are a good communicator. Tissue is skin or gum or whatever organ you may be treating. By watching for body language you may pick up on moments when patients don't understand and you can slow down or explain over again when necessary.

––––––––––––

There was this couple whose husband experienced the loss of libido. Upon returning from the doctor he entered the house wearing a tuxedo. His wife asked anxiously if he had seen the doctor about his problem. "Of course!" he replied.

"Well, why are you all dressed up in a tuxedo?" she queried.

"The doctor said I'm impotent, so if I'm impotent, I figured I should look impotent."

––––––––––––

There are many words that should be stricken from your vocabulary when speaking with patients. Here are some examples and proper ways to say the same thing.

Avoid using the term "incision." Instead tell your patients **"I will make a small opening"**

I&D means nothing to most patients, however, they understand, **"We are going to release the pressure."**

Going under the knife? Can you sound any more barbaric? Try, **"You need a surgical procedure."**

Purulent drainage is **pus** to the layman. Use their language.

Who knows what a patient might think when you tell them you are laying a flap? It is much more comprehensible to tell them you are going to **"pull back"** the gum, skin or whatever you are operating upon.

Curetting is **clean out**, enucleating is **removing**, and an exploratory operation sounds much better if it is described simply as you **"are going to look around."**

The term "prognosis" is used all the time. Stop using it with your patients. **"The chance of this working out"** is much easier to understand. Yes, there are patients who have no idea what prognosis means, and they are too embarrassed to ask.

Sure, you didn't go to medical school to speak like an idiot, but you have to communicate to your patients in a clear, non-threatening manner if you want to have the best bedside manner.

It is a great idea to get a small digital recorder and listen to at least a dozen of your presentations of treatment plans or explaining procedures. You may be surprised at how you sound to your patients.

Despite your best efforts, there are some patients who will never fully understand your explanation of a complex procedure. To offer the best possible service and chance of success, you should always have **written instructions** for each procedure you perform.

Written instructions are a wonderful way to enhance the way you communicate with your patients. While some patients don't understand anything you tell them, never read your instructions, and are not very compliant because of their lack of understanding and lack of interest, there are those who appreciate the written word.

WRITTEN COMMUNICATIONS – THE HANDOUTS

Written handouts are a simple way to communicate more effectively with your patients, and they require no personality or social skills on your part, as do oral communications.

Besides enhancing your bedside manner by utilizing good communication skills, **written handouts**, **diagrams** used in explaining procedures, and **signed consent forms** will help keep you out of the courtroom. Most plaintiffs' attorneys won't take a case when they see great documentation and the damages are not significant. Even if you end up in court, it is very difficult for the plaintiff to convince a jury of laymen that you didn't explain anything when it's all there in black and white.

At minimum, every practitioner should have a **written informed consent** carefully constructed with the advice of a professional organization or an attorney versed in such matters, a **pamphlet describing what you do in lay terms** and what to expect from treatment, and a **post treatment instruction sheet** that includes what to expect and how to handle after hours emergencies.

The post treatment instructions are especially important. Rather than calling you in the middle of the night, your patients can read the directions if they experience complications after they leave your office.

If your procedures require multiple visits, make sure you give the patient the post treatment instruction sheet after each visit. While you may think patients save your instruction sheet in a scrapbook of important documents to be passed on to their heirs, they usually throw them away. By handing patients a sheet of instructions after each visit, they will have help when they need it.

People generally remember first and last impressions. To become the great doctor everyone wants to see, always leave your patients on a positive note. When you dismiss your patients, always give them reassurance: "If there's anything you don't understand or need help with later, don't hesitate to give us a call." This reassurance is the ultimate form of communication in that it tells your patients they can get answers to anything they didn't understand. Knowing you are there for them goes a long way toward having a meaningful doctor-patient relationship.

Patients getting a second opinion will almost always choose the doctor who explains things better. If you're the first opinion and have great communication skills, most patients won't even consider getting a second opinion.

COMMUNICATING FINANCIAL ISSUES

Financial considerations are one of the biggest reasons patients get upset with their doctors. If you want a distinguished reputation, besides being compassionate in handling fiscal matters as described in the chapter on compassion, you must communicate fees and expectations for payment.

Most patients expect insurance companies to pay for services and when unexpected co-payments arise they often get upset. Just because your forms state that patients are responsible for any unpaid fees, patients may claim they didn't see, read, or understand the notice.

A well-trained front desk is the key to avoid misunderstandings. They should present financial expectations at the initial call after setting up the appointment. Your staff should have the means to check insurance coverage by phone or Internet connection. They should emphasize that any co-payment they quote is only an estimate based on the "information you provided."

Many patients believe doctors are wealthy and cannot understand how healing arts professionals could possibly ask them to pay the meager ten-dollar co-payment. They usually have little understanding of reimbursement schedules requiring doctors to treat patients for minimal fees that at times don't pay for overhead costs. Well-scripted employees can respond to the cynical patient commenting on why the doctor "really needs my ten dollars."

"Mr. Jones, in order to participate with your insurance company and provide you and your family with the best of care, Dr. Smith accepts greatly reduced fees. Your insurance company determines the co-payment, not the doctor, and that helps to supplement the reduced fees. Between insurance company payments and your co-payment, it doesn't leave much profit for many of the procedures Dr. Smith performs. I do hope you can understand we are trying to keep payment by the patient as low as possible by participating with these insurance plans. That's why we have to collect these modest co-payments."

No matter how wonderful your bedside manner, if the patient can't afford the bill, thinks they were charged more than they were told upon initial contact, or feels their financial responsibility wasn't explained appropriately, they will not come back to see you. Quite often, they will badmouth you to validate their perception of injustice.

If your practice deals with emergency care, you may not have the luxury of obtaining preauthorization, in which case you may want to estimate patient financial responsibility and have the patient sign a statement indicating that until the insurance coverage can be verified, they will be responsible for any unpaid charges.

If you withhold care for financial reasons, make sure you offer a less expensive alternative. Patients will not perceive you as compassionate (or worthy of being called a doctor), if money is your only consideration for providing service.

Some patients perceive any discussion of money as unprofessional. Try to avoid placing undue emphasis on financial matters. On initial contact by phone, bring up fees and financial arrangements *after* attending to all of the patient's questions concerning treatment and making an appointment. Fees should always be discussed but not at the first moment of contact.

Even in cases where the patient has no co-payments, they may be jealous and have disdain for doctors when they see how much they are paid for various procedures. The days of appreciating the skills of a great doctor are being replaced by a world of envious people wanting to consume more than they contribute. This attitude is all the more reason for healthcare professionals to be clear about financial matters.

COMMUNICATING WITH YOUR STAFF

Communicating with your staff is just as important as communicating with your patients. And how your staff communicates with the patients is equally important. Besides assuring that they assist you in the appropriate manner while performing technical procedures, they can help explain routine things and answer common questions with your prepared, fully scripted responses.

Make sure your staff understands every procedure you perform, but don't let them explain or respond to complex or controversial questions. The last thing you need is a patient making claims that your nurse told them something for which you could be liable.

Your staff should never give medical advice. This happens in many offices in spite of the potential risks. Every time a staff member tells a patient what to do regarding postoperative care, it could be perceived of as medical advice. That is why it is important that you clearly instruct your staff with appropriate scripting anytime you have them give patient instructions.

Your staff should not be instructing patients on issues like dosage of medication unless you have a standing protocol that doesn't necessitate that they ask you in each case. For example, if patients call with continued swelling that may require doubling the dosage of an antibiotic or anti-inflammatory agent, and you routinely make that recommendation, you may allow your staff to make that recommendation without asking you. Of course make sure they get the appropriate information about the patient's condition and document the conversation in the patient chart. You must be able to justify the recommendation when a savvy personal injury attorney tells a jury that you should have spoken with the patient and should have never let your staff make the recommendation.

There are so many instances where we let staff communicate instructions to the patient that we take for granted. Having a secretary tell the patient to use hot compresses or ice or any other recommendation must be grounded in sound practice. This requires more instruction than allowing staff to make the recommendation they heard you make a hundred times unless that recommendation is the only appropriate option.

You don't want to have to defend yourself in a case where your secretary told a patient to place a hot compress on an abdominal pain that turns into a burst appendix, just because they heard you make that recommendation for some other ailment.

Every area of practice has certain routine recommendations that are offered to the patient on the phone every day. While it is best for you to make all the decisions, practically speaking, you do have to delegate certain duties. Make sure you have documented that you trained each staff member regarding any recommendations you have them make. This is best written into a staff manual. Naturally, any recommendation made by your staff should be documented in the patient chart with your initials.

An Endodontist Says:
When patients call with postoperative pain, I have my
secretary ask a few key questions:
"Is there any swelling? Do you feel feverish? Does it hurt
to close your teeth together without
any food in your mouth?"

As long as they respond "no" to those questions, I have
my secretary use the following script:

"I want you to rinse your mouth with hot saltwater for five minutes each hour. You can take the pain medicine prescribed if the Advil or Tylenol doesn't help. If there is no change in twenty-four hours I'd like you to call back and let me know."

This way, I know there is consistency in communicating the appropriate instructions to the patient. If they are swelling or have any fever, or if they can't bite down, I want them to come in to see me.

Each realm of treatment requires that you prepare scripts as described above and make sure anything that can be confusing is not left for the front desk to handle.

If the patient insists on speaking with the doctor, your policy should provide for them to speak with the doctor. While you can't be expected to stop everything to speak with patients when it is not practical, you should set up a system that encourages the patient to work out their problem with the front desk. Perhaps a policy like this may help:

Dr. Jones is with patients and can't come to the phone this moment. If you would like to tell me your problem, I may be able to help you, or relay your message to Dr. Jones so we can see you today if necessary."

If the patient is insistent, proceed:

"I'll be happy to have Dr. Jones call you back when he is finished with patients or sooner if he gets a break. That usually is at the end of his appointment hours, so if I can help you regarding any emergency concerns, it would be best to tell me now. That way we can get you in today if necessary. Otherwise I will have him call you as soon as possible. If he calls you after hours, he won't be able to see you today, so please let me help you now."

This script offers the patient two chances to work with the front desk staff. It let's them know you won't necessarily be calling them back until after hours. It tells them that emergency questions should be mentioned at that moment if they expect to come in to see the doctor that day. And it is not refusing their request to speak with the doctor.

There are some doctors who take patient calls as they come through. While that is not an easy task, it sure makes the patients on the phone happy, while the ones being treated may not be overjoyed by multiple interruptions. You decide.

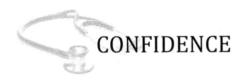

CONFIDENCE

The goal of seeking out healthcare is to resolve one problem or another. Who wouldn't want to see the very best, most *competent* practitioner around? How can the image of competence be better portrayed than through exuding **confidence**?

A Dental Specialist Says
I get to see the quality of many practitioners' work. The most interesting phenomenon about how many doctors are perceived by their patients is through the confidence they exhibit. I know two fellows in particular who had enormous practices and their patients' loved them even though they may have been the most incompetent guys I ever knew. What they excelled in was confidence. It was unbelievable how many of their patients thought they were with the best doctor around.

Since competence and confidence are not always paired together as they should be, we must recognize that the purpose of this discourse is not to fool the unsuspecting public by explaining how to express confidence. It is however incumbent upon every practitioner to have the utmost confidence in everything they do to improve their bedside manner and to provide the finest possible experience for each and every patient.

Even the effectiveness of **placebo** has been shown in studies to be enhanced by the confidence/bedside manner of the practitioner. In The Annals of Internal Medicine, 4 June 2002, Vol.136, pg. 817-825, authors Eisenberg and Kaptchuk discuss the performance of **"healing ritual"** as part of the patient-practitioner interaction and how it may affect healing. As practitioners, we have an obligation to make sure our "rituals" are filled with compassion and confidence, as they not only build our reputation and practice, they may actually help to heal our patients.

The best way to have confidence is to know your field to the nth degree. Be able to answer every question posed to you. And when you don't know the answer, make sure it is because *no one* knows the answer. No one wants to go to the doctor who can't answer their questions or the one who stammers or seems stumped by the questions and has to contemplate the answers. If you truly know your field of practice, and have been doing it long enough, you probably heard most every question that could be thought up and that is where experience helps.

It is interesting how the *confident, incompetent* practitioners seem to be able to answer all the questions even when they don't know the *right* answers. The reason lies in the fact that they quite often give the wrong answer with such confidence that they are never questioned further or second guessed. Since their patients love and trust them, they don't often get second opinions. They are not inclined to seek redress when things go wrong.

Besides knowing your field like no one else, you have to convey your confidence to the patient. Remember, there are some exceptionally talented and bright practitioners who have such poor bedside manner that if someone didn't tell the patients that this doctor is the best, no one would go there.

CONVEYING CONFIDENCE

To convey confidence you have to be a good communicator and that is why communication ties in so well as one of the bedrocks of bedside manner. Confident communicators offer all the information necessary for the patient to feel they are making an appropriate choice in their selection of "you" and the procedure you recommend.

When offering treatment options, make sure you have an opinion about that which is best. The confident doctor is not afraid to guide the patient. The last thing you want to appear is wishy-washy. Guiding the patient doesn't preclude your responsibility to offer all options of treatment as part of the informed consent, it just means that you aren't afraid to tell the patient what you think is best.

A Patient's Story
I needed to have back surgery and I went to this one guy who told me it would definitely help and that he too needed to have the same surgery. He then told me, "In truth, I'm afraid to get it done, and I keep putting it off." Naturally, I went for a second opinion, especially because I could barely walk. The next guy was very direct. He told me I definitely needed the surgery and even showed me how my leg was getting weaker and the muscle was shrinking. He told me that he had it done and is doing fine. He did warn me of the downside consequences, but clearly stated that doing nothing in my case was more of a risk for permanent problems. The thing I liked best and sold me on him was when he said, "You don't have to get this done by me, but you need to get it done." I schedule right then to have it done the next week, No need for any more opinions for me.

Looking directly at the patient when you speak is a good trait for communicating and even more important in expressing confidence. Confident people don't look down at the floor. Naturally there are times you are writing notes in a chart, or looking over reports and x-rays. That is not the time to discuss the case with the patient. Put down your pen and step away from the view box. Move the reports to the side. When you speak to your patient pay close attention and engage them with your eyes.

Have your pitch well rehearsed. Make sure it answers all the questions you've heard a thousand times. If the patient is sharp and has no questions by the time you are done, you have communicated well and in a most confident manner. If you really excel, don't be surprised if patients keep asking questions and encourage other conversation because they are so delighted with your manner and presentation.

There are two ways to convey confidence. One couples with compassion while the other couples with authoritarianism. Both work with differing personalities. Some patients like to put their doctors on pedestals and actually feel good when the doctor speaks in an affirmative manner. Picture the older doctor looking down so his eyes peer above bifocals balanced on the tip of his nose as he delivers his directives.

Others prefer the doctor whose confidence is built into a deeper level of compassion. This doctor can speak softly and slowly in a manner that exudes confidence with the *compassionate touch*. Each practitioner has to exhibit that type of confidence that best suits his personality and taste.

YOUR REPUTATION

An indirect way of engendering confidence in your patients takes place before they walk in your door. This occurs as a result of your reputation. Patients often rely on recommendations from friends, family, and especially other professionals. Everyone likes to go to "the best" and when they hear the same name popup time and again, they have confidence before they even meet with you. Never take your reputation for granted and never miss the opportunity to develop it. Be a great doctor and the word spreads.

The Secretary
We're referring you to Dr. Jones. He is amaz-
ing. He treated me and my husband. As a mat-
ter of fact, he treated Dr. Smith too, and that's
why he sends all his patients to Dr. Jones.

There used to be a concept in healthcare called **professional courtesy**. It was a common, unwritten rule that doctors would treat each other without fees. This practice has dried up in many instances. It seems that everyone wants to make a lot of money and they don't consider how offering colleagues a courtesy may be appropriate.

There is one bastion of professional courtesy that remains, and that is providing free care for those who refer patients to you. It has become a matter of quid pro quo today with the expected gain associated with catering to your source of patients.

It is sad that so many behaviors are associated with self-interest. It is wise to at least know that professional courtesy for your referring doctors as well as their family and staff members means they will generally be loyal to you. When they recommend you and tell their patient how great you are, it becomes an immediate endorsement that goes a long way in enhancing your reputation even though it may have nothing to do with your abilities.

If you treat your patients with all the pillars of great bedside manner and you are truly great at what you do, your reputation will grow without relying on who you treat for free. Then you can offer professional courtesy because it may just be the right thing to do.

CONFIDENCE IN THE FACE OF ADVERSITY

Confidence is needed more than ever when things go wrong. There are certain risks with most every treatment modality in every field of practice. Instruments break, tissues don't always heal, and treatments fail. Things don't always go well.

You must rehearse your explanations of untoward results and present them with confidence. This way you will have less negative repercussions.

When an instrument breaks, it is much better to have a sound, logical explanation and solution that you present with all the confidence that portrays the event as something within the realm of reasonable possibilities. Contrasted with a panicky presentation that tells the patient you messed up; confidence wins every time.

Areas of adversity differ with each field of practice. If you deal with life and death issues, you must have a script for telling loved ones that the patient died. A lesser case of adversity may deal with a failed procedure. The more important the procedure, the more difficult the explanation may become. It is much easier to tell the patient the scar on their back isn't fading than telling the patient the heart transplant failed, however, no matter how trivial the loss, **compassion** must remain a constant.

No matter how trivial you may value any adversity, every case warrants a good, and especially confident explanation for why things didn't work out as planned. The **informed consent** that specifically explains many of the complications of treatment helps make your explanation of a failing procedure that much more acceptable. And when delivered compassionately and with great confidence, the patient is more likely to accept the outcome.

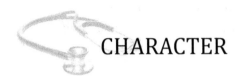

CHARACTER

All kinds of people choose the healing arts, just like any other field of endeavor. Some of them are unsavory characters and some just make bad choices in critical areas of their lives. Patients expect a higher level of behavior from those to whom they entrust their care.

The research a medical doctor performed for a major drug company was called into question after he was arrested on his front lawn, brandishing a gun, naked except for underwear that hid his cocaine along with his private parts.

An orthodontist was convicted of molesting young girls and went to prison. Because he lost his license and could no longer work, he applied for disability insurance. Denied.

A popular pain center became a haven for drug abusers to get prescriptions for hundreds of narcotic painkillers. The doctor was discovered and sent to prison.

The doctor spent countless hours in the office; the hectic schedule of practice took a great toll on his marital relationship. Pretty soon the doctor found staying late at work was better than the constant harassment at home. The office manager soon became his love interest and eventually the wife of the unsettled practitioner.

Stories like these are played out in too many lives, and there are many other areas in which character flaws ruin the lives of health-care providers. Substance abuse and insurance fraud have destroyed many careers. Without question, these criminal acts are reprehensible. Reputation is tainted and ability to continue in professional practice becomes doubtful. Fortunately, not too many health-care professionals act out criminal behaviors. Those who engage in such activities should be removed from the system.

There are moral lapses that won't land you in prison, but that will deeply affect reputation. While character may not appear to be a component of bedside manner, it is most definitely an integral factor. Sex and money are the two biggest areas of ethical and moral conflict.

It's easy to fall prey to your ego and the power that comes with your position. Making inappropriate advances to patients or accepting such advances puts you in jeopardy. If you have affairs with patients, you risk losing your spouse (if you have one), your license, your wealth and your dignity. If you must fulfill sexual needs, do it outside of your office.

Involvement with staff has ruined many marriages and once-successful practices. It is easy to succumb to desire when you work many hours away from home. Staff who may admire you or are searching for wealth and station afforded by professional association can often entice you towards unethical conduct. It is best to keep your professional relations at a distance and avoid too much informality.

You can be a great salesman and have a fabulous bedside manner, but if you sell things the patient doesn't need or can't afford, you lack ethics. The area of cosmetic practice lends itself to such abuse with the promise of even better results if you only consider this other procedure. Prolonging treatment for months beyond necessity in order to drag out payment makes patients question your integrity.

An unhappy patient: "After feeling completely improved, the doctor told me I needed to continue having the adjustments. When I asked him when I would be able to stop, he told me that to maintain my good health I should consider having these adjustments throughout my life. I never went back."

The astute patient may discover billing for procedures that weren't performed when they show up on insurance statements. While some patients may believe their best interest is at heart, others will have a justifiable loss of trust. In time, most practitioners who put sales above need and income above integrity are discovered.

If your staff respects you and values their employment, their admiration projects to the patients. By attracting and retaining great staff, your practice runs better and time spent training new hires is greatly reduced. Disgruntled employees should be weeded out and dismissed. There is nothing more counterproductive to developing a great bedside manner than to be surrounded by people who undermine it by speaking negatively about the doctor, and being miserable, curt, or aloof to patients.

Pay your staff a fair wage and provide good benefits. Be fair in resolving disputes between staff members and between staff and patients when a conflict arises. Never berate staff or talk to them in a condescending manner. If they are so inept that you feel the necessity to scold them, they should be dismissed. Treat all of your team with respect and dignity.

Don't forget your staff on holidays (Christmas, Valentine's Day, Secretaries' Day, and Assistants' Day). Flowers, candy, a tray of cookies, tickets to the movies or theater, and even an office outing go a long way toward showing appreciation for the people who help make your life better. Treating your staff well is all part of your character and relates to your bedside manner.

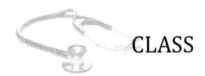 CLASS

A woman went to the doctor's office. She was seen by one of the new doctors, but after about 4 minutes in the examination room, she burst out, screaming as she ran down the hall. An older doctor stopped and asked her what the problem was, and she explained. He had her sit down and relax in another room.

The older doctor marched back to the first and demanded, "What's the matter with you? Mrs. Johnson is 65 years old, she has four grown children and seven grandchildren, and you told her she was pregnant?" The new doctor smiled smugly as he continued to write on his clipboard.

"Cured her hiccups though, didn't it?"

Class encompasses the way you speak, conduct yourself, and your appearance. Many doctors don't realize how these factors are important components of their bedside manner.

The more your patient population relates with you–while you maintain professional stature–the more you will be liked. Appearance and language change from one locale to another and constantly evolve with societal mores and styles. The longer you practice, the more likely you need to change, in order to keep current with how society defines a professional.

The following story relates to a practitioner who has no class and no compassion when speaking with patients.

———————

A renowned oncologic head and neck surgeon saw a patient of mine diagnosed with stage four tonsilar cancer. This doctor was physically intimidating; a very tall man with an in-your-face posture. Furthermore, he was demeaning, cold, and inconsiderate of the patient's feelings. When he presented his protocol of treatment, he told the patient there was no one who could do the surgery as well as he could, and that if the patient didn't go along with his treatment, "You will die a horrible painful death." The patient, also being a rather large, intimidating man, got into his face and told him there was no way he would want to use him as a doctor. Interestingly, I had the opportunity to treat a nurse on the oncologist's service, and I asked her if she could tell me anything about this doctor. She made a face of disgust and asked me why I made such an inquiry. When I relayed the story of the terrified patient, she stated that this doctor speaks that way to all of his patients. She confirmed that he was probably the best surgeon in the area for this procedure and that is why she suspected the hospital kept him on staff. She further stated that he not only had no bedside manner, but that he was the antithesis of the concept. She was so riled by the thought of this man that she asked me if I would write a letter to the hospital administrator relaying the story I told to her.

———————

It is best to do a demographic review of your patient population. Demographics describe populations according to age, income, product preferences, and just about any measurable attribute, including health-care needs.

By utilizing demographic information, you can know what kind of conversation patients will enjoy, what marketing to consider, what type of magazines to include in your waiting room, and even what channel to keep on the television in the waiting room at different times of the day.

The Elderly (55 +)

Past generations get stuck in time. You have to remember this when dealing with the elderly. Elderly patients tend to be more conservative, they are respectful, and many deride the latest styles of the young. This is the population you need to think about before you become a trailblazer of pop-culture as defined by your fashion and language. Your senior patients won't respond well to hip-hop music playing in the waiting room or dress unbefitting their perception of a professional.

The way you address and speak with the elderly is clearly different from the way you deal with younger people. Seniors may be offended if you call them by first name or if you introduce yourself by your first name. This is the generation that puts doctors on pedestals and demands professionalism, as defined years ago. These are the patients who expect that you have answers to their questions and that you will not rush them during an examination.

The Youth (15 – 25)

If you treat many young patients, you will relate better and be perceived as having better bedside manner if you throw in a few slang phrases. However, you must be careful. Just because you may treat many young people, your elderly patients seldom embrace the slang and values of the younger set and may be offended.

If you see a young patient and wish to connect in an informal manner, you can alter your greeting to, "Hey, what's up?" While this may not be your usual greeting, it could, in this instance, form an immediate bond of trust.

No one will fault you for not using slang. Ironically, many youthful patients may actually question your expertise if you speak and act like them. Remember, you can never offend someone by being polite and well spoken.

Try not to take offense by the way patients speak to you. It's usually not personal. The aggressive talk of a person brought up in a bravado culture is part of their personality and not likely to change at a visit with the doctor. Some patients are frightened or stressed and may react in a coarse or belligerent manner. Of course there are some patients who are hostile and their behavior doesn't have to be tolerated.

Upper Crust

Many successful, professional, or upwardly mobile patients like to claim personal friendships with their health-care providers. Some will insist on calling you by your first name and want to become friends with you. You have to make the decision how to react to what, at times, may be intrusive.

This type of patient may drop first names of other professionals giving the impression they are personal friends; and while they may be, they may be using the names to get more attention and reduced fees.

Generally speaking, if a patient calls me by my first name or asks if I mind, I have no problem going along with them. If you tell them you prefer that they call you by your title, you might be perceived as stuffy.

Some doctors like to introduce themselves by first name believing it enhances bedside manner by being more personal. I prefer to maintain a professional stature that is warm and friendly rather than trying to be my patients' best friend. It is best not to encourage personal relationships with patients or you may find an examination or treatment visit turn into a social call. Furthermore, there is something more authoritative about following the directions of the doctor rather than a buddy.

A busy neurologist: "Every time I see neighbors or friends in the office, they never seem to understand how behind I get when they decide to ask about my family and my life, and they then proceed to tell me about their family and life. I can't be rude, but I surely couldn't practice if I became friends with all my patients. It's one thing to be friendly and ask about family in a controlled manner, but too much familiarity is not a good thing."

GROOMING

Grooming is important to the way patients perceive their doctors. If a patient sees a poorly groomed practitioner, it doesn't take much to extend the lack of grooming to a possible lack of professionalism and competence and especially cleanliness. We all know that long dirty hair, bad breath, and soiled fingernails don't necessarily mean you aren't a capable doctor–but most people would rather go to a doctor who understands and respects the necessity of proper grooming.

Most people want a well-groomed, well-mannered doctor. Personal hygiene is imperative.

Hygiene Don'ts:

- Bad Breath

Avoid eating onions, garlic, peppers or any foods that repeat on you for lunch or dinner the preceding evening. Consider chewing a mint-flavored gum throughout the day. Use the gum more as a lozenge to avoid visible chewing motion. If you have a noticeable, longstanding problem with bad breath there are intensive programs available to help you.

- Hair

Hair should be worn in an acceptable, conservative style. You don't have to have a crew cut or a bun, but extreme styles should be avoided. The times dictate style. A beard and longer hair for men are more acceptable at certain times in history. The best rule is to avoid being at the leading edge. If no one wears beards then you should refrain. If everyone is wearing a day's growth of beard, it may be acceptable. Just don't be the trailblazer.

If you have a bushel of chest or back hair growing out of your scrubs, trim it.

Conversation of staff members about one of the doctors: "I can't believe how gross he looks with that hair billowing out of his scrubs. He is completely oblivious!"

Make sure you don't have hair growing out of your ears or nose to any appreciable degree.

- Other Issues

Your fingernails should always be clean and well trimmed.

If you have oily skin, do regular checks and wipe or cleanse your face as needed. Check for wax or flaking skin in your ears.

Brush your teeth after meals and look in a mirror to make sure you don't have food stuck between your teeth when you speak with your patients.

If you have a bad acne condition, seek the appropriate care.

Try to remedy any postnasal drip sounds and assorted tics that may be undesirable. Constantly clearing your throat may be a turnoff to some patients.

Avoid strong colognes and perfumes.

If you perspire heavily, keep a change of shirts or blouses in your office and use them as needed.

Make sure you have someone on your staff you can trust to call your attention to things like body odor. If you have the proper rapport, they will know you trust their critique, and they will be able to tell you when something is amiss. You cannot afford to be complacent about how you present yourself to your patients. Grooming and work habits matter.

ATTIRE

It is imperative for you to maintain attire befitting a learned practitioner – even on your days off. If country clubs can require a collared shirt, you can wear one when you go to the hardware store to purchase plumbing parts for your home repairs. If you want to have the consummate reputation and the ultimate bedside manner, you have to dress the part. You never know who you might bump into.

Can you picture a patient seeing you at the hardware store looking like a bum and turning to their best friend to rave about you? While your patient may see past your attire, their friend will respond, "He's a doctor?"

Rules for Dressing Appropriately

Pants should be clean and pressed. Business trousers or khakis are acceptable, but if you are looking for a more polished look, consider seamed trousers. A smock or clean, white pressed doctor's jacket goes best with pants. Scrubs are a casual and more comfortable choice, but they too must be clean and presentable. The suit and tie says something special for consultation office visits.

Leather shoes are traditional and they must be polished and devoid of any signs of excessive wear. If you prefer athletic shoes to go with scrubs, make sure they are clean – save a pair for the office and don't use them for jogging.

For women who prefer skirts and blouses, suits or dresses, too-short hemlines and obvious cleavage should be avoided.

When I attended dental school, the style was long hair, bell-bottom pants, and open shirts with bead necklaces. While we thought we were cool and nonconformist, the older population of patients thought we were arrogant, inconsiderate, and unprofessional.

I worked for an older doctor during those hippie days while many of my friends opened their offices wearing jeans and long wild hair styles. When my new employer told me I had to wear a dress shirt and tie (these were the days before scrubs and masks), I was mortified. How was I ever to express my individualism and flourish among the flower children? I went along with his request because I needed the job.

When I opened my own specialty practice that relied upon referrals from other doctors, I realized that I couldn't offend anyone if I wore a shirt and tie. None of my patients could go back to their doctors and complain that I wore a shirt and tie.

Some of my referring doctors were hippies and wore the bell-bottoms and open shirts, but my best referrers were older established doctors who wore clinic gowns and conservative hairstyles. While I may not have been the coolest endodontist, I built up a great practice with referrals from my hippie friends as well as all of the established dentists who would never refer their patients to a hippie.

Making staff wear presentable attire never leads to rumors that your office is unprofessional. Your staff is a reflection of your personality. Poorly groomed or poorly dressed staff doesn't belong in anyone's office.

The same principle of trying to avoid offending anyone applies to the music you play in your office. Referring to the demographic of my patient population, I found that most of my patients were between forty and sixty years of age. As a group, they don't generally appreciate heavy metal or hip-hop music. Surprisingly, some popular radio stations that tout playing a blend of tunes with the intention of appealing to everyone always seem to air some terribly inappropriate songs that are offensive to that age group. Make sure the music you play in your office won't offend anyone.

VOICE

A truly unrecognized attribute of demeanor is the volume and tone of voice, which can range from soft and calming to loud and irritating.

You can adjust your voice to meet the needs of various patients. Many nervous patients love a soft calming voice when offering explanations and during treatment. You can't go wrong with soft and calming–but too soft and inaudible is not good, especially for the elderly.

Your loud and outgoing patients will connect with you if you, too, are animated and loud. You must know your patients, but generally try to stay away from loud and boisterous.

Being outgoing, cheerful, jocular, and personable is almost universally appreciated, so strive for those traits without being too over-the-top.

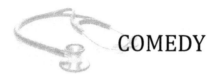

COMEDY

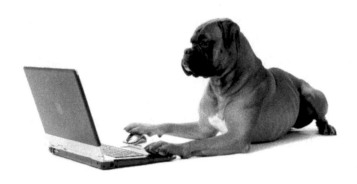

It was entertainment night at the senior center. The amazing Claude was appearing that night and the crowd waited anxiously to see the famed hypnotist. When Claude came to the stage, he announced, "Unlike most hypnotists who invite two or three people from the audience to come up and get put into a trance, I intend to hypnotize each and every member of the audience." He removed a beautiful antique watch from his coat pocket and said, "I want each and every one of you to keep your eye on this antique watch. It's a very special watch. It has been in my family for six generations." He began to swing the watch back and forth while quietly chanting, "Watch the watch, watch the watch, watch the watch..." The crowd was mesmerized as they

watched the light gleaming off of the bright shiny object. All eyes followed the swaying watch when all of a sudden it slipped from the amazing Claude's fingers, fell to the floor and shattered into a hundred pieces.

"Crap!" said the hypnotist...
It took three days to clean up the senior center.

The anatomy of comedy finds its essence in the absurd, the ironic, the exaggerated, and the unexpected. The main purpose of comedy is to make us laugh, but it often teaches us lessons, and more importantly, it connects people together in a manner that engenders likeability. Laughter is a priceless involuntary response to visual and/or verbal stimuli.

Everyone loves to laugh and be around funny people. Who doesn't like a good joke? Humor is the greatest technique for easing the fearful patient, disarming the belligerent patient, and making all of your patients like you.

You don't have to have been the class clown or the most personable individual to succeed with using humor. Memorizing jokes that you wouldn't have time to tell in a busy practice is not necessary. Effective comedy can be learned. There are simple lines that work well most of the time.

Most jokes involve two parts: the set up and the punch line. A pause is often used in delivering comedic lines for its ability to magnify the punch line. The difference between a chuckle and a hearty laugh can often be attributed to the proper use of the pause. It's called timing.

There are some people who are morbidly unhappy, miserable, or otherwise without any sense of humor. They may be depressed, involved in bad relationships, having a bad day, or they may have never learned to appreciate the joys of comedy. Humor is also cultural, so patients from other countries may not always get your jokes or humorous comments. Don't get discouraged if you use a line from this text and you get a blank stare. Keep trying and you will soon realize you are actually funny.

There are those gifted people for whom a big part of their comedic talent is spontaneous. These are the people we consider funny, not by virtue of memorized lines or reciting formal jokes. These are the people who have a talent for finding humor in things happening at the moment and being able to comment on them instantaneously – they can improvise. Don't expect to learn how to do this here. That kind of talent takes a special type of brain. Instead, you can learn to deliver funny lines specifically prepared for health-care providers. Once you get the hang of it, you can improvise and customize lines for your practice.

You can learn to deliver funny lines even if others have described you as being a dullard. Just like you learned the Krebs cycle, you can learn to deliver a few select lines. To become proficient you will need to study and practice your newfound skills. You have to use the skills regularly or you will forget them, just like you forgot the Krebs cycle. Once you see how effective humor works, you will never go back to being a boring health-care provider.

If the patient gives you a funny look or if they react in an odd manner to any of your comedy lines don't be afraid to tell them you are "just kidding." "Just kidding" confirms that you are a joker and allays any fears felt by patients who either have no sense of humor or who may not get the joke. If the occasional patient doesn't appreciate your humor, back off and let them experience a bland visit.

GREETINGS

The first impression is often the most important. Upon entering the room, you have the opportunity to establish how you will be perceived in the professional relationship. In these thirty seconds you can ease tension, dispel fears, show your humanity, and engender affection.

If you begin by mumbling, "Morning," you will be perceived, at best, as a quiet reserved practitioner and, at worst, as an unfriendly

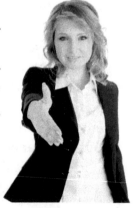

burnt-out practitioner. If you enter the room and begin by announcing in a friendly, almost singing, tone, "Good morning, and how are you doing today?" you will be perceived as a friendly, outgoing, happy person. Patients prefer the affable approach to the withdrawn, almost miserable overture.

The introduction is the most important moment of bonding. No matter how warm and friendly you greet the new patient; it doesn't come close to the positive impact achieved by being able to make them laugh. Your main objective is to make your patient, at minimum, smile and, at best, laugh within thirty seconds.

Begin your greeting in the very expected manner: "Good morning, how are you doing today?"

You must always know what to expect when you ask any question, and with the greeting there are only three general responses you will hear. The patient is either good, bad, or they say nothing. While "no response" from your patient is not typical, it happens on occasion and you have to be ready for anything coming your way.

No Response from the Patient

If you are a psychiatrist treating catatonic patients you can stop with your initial greeting, make some observational notes in the chart, walk out of the room, and bill the State for a comprehensive exam. Assuming your patient isn't comatose, you can respond to the silent patient:

DOCTOR
"Good morning and how are you doing, today?"

PATIENT
No response.

DOCTOR
"It's okay. You can talk to me. I don't charge by the word."

Variation:
"I guess you're not doing so well or you'd tell me you were fine and I would let you leave."

Variation:
"I don't need much from you, just name, rank, and serial number."

Variation:
"Okay, how about them Yankees?"

The patient will usually respond to any of these lines, realizing you expected an answer. Don't worry if the patient doesn't laugh, because people who don't say hello usually don't laugh either, and people who are frightened may expectedly not respond. You can't make everyone laugh; don't take it personally. Many times the unresponsive patient is either frightened, in pain, or shy. By joking around, they will often warm up. The chapter on body language contains more on managing the unresponsive patient.

Patient Is Feeling Fine

Getting back to greeting the patient who is feeling fine:

DOCTOR
"Good morning and how are you doing today?"

PATIENT
"Fine."

DOCTOR
"Fine? Then what are you doing here?"

Ninety percent of your patients are going to smile or laugh. This ninety percent now likes you, and if you keep up the routine they will love you by the time they are ready to leave.

The patient may respond to your initial greeting with:

PATIENT
"I'm fine doctor. How are you?"

Don't let this variation on the theme throw you for a loop. It's really quite simple, you say:

DOCTOR
"I'm doing well, too."

Pause:

"If we're both so good, what are we doing here?"

Variation after the pause:

DOCTOR
"We're both doing fine, it's a nice day; let's get out of this place."

Bingo! They smile or laugh.

When the patient is fine, you have an opportunity to use another line that gets a great response. You now query them about things like symptoms and their current condition.

DOCTOR
"Are you having any pain?"

PATIENT
"No."

DOCTOR
"Well, I can fix that."

You can use this line if the patient says they are fine as in the first example, too. This makes most patients laugh. If they don't, just keep telling yourself it isn't you, and you'll be fine.

Pause just a bit after their chuckle, and proceed:

DOCTOR
"As a matter of fact, that's my specialty!"

You now own this patient. They will never leave you unless they find out you don't accept their insurance.

Patient Is Feeling Bad

DOCTOR
"So, how are you doing this fine afternoon?"

PATIENT
"Terrible!"

The patient may elaborate:

PATIENT TWO
"I'm not doing so well. I was up all night in pain."

From this response, the astute practitioner should immediately realize this patient needs their help, even if they don't accept the patient's insurance.

DOCTOR
"Gee, I was hoping one of us was feeling okay."

Variation for patient two:

DOCTOR
"Then you're in the right place. All day long, I see people who were up all night and *most* of them survive this experience."

Assuming the patient isn't in acute pain, they will smile. Don't expect the laugh. If they are in true distress you will want to hold up on the humor, as it may seem unsympathetic.

Sometimes you encounter the SARCASTIC PATIENT:

DOCTOR
"Good morning and how are you today?"

PATIENT
"If I was that good, I wouldn't be here."

DOCTOR
"Well, I'm doing *great* and I'm here.
One of us must be in the wrong place."

This line helps to disarm the sarcastic patient, and it let's them see you have a sense of humor.

The Patient with a Companion

When you enter the treatment room and find a spouse or other adult friend accompanying the patient who is seated on the examination table or treatment chair, say:

DOCTOR
"Good morning. How's everyone doing today?"

You will get an answer from one or both of the parties. As long as they don't burst into explaining why they are there (some patients and their guests impulsively want to tell you their story before you ask), you look at the visitor and say:

DOCTOR
"I suppose you're the patient and you talked Jim, here, into sitting in that chair, so you could find out what we're going to do to you."

Unless the couple doesn't speak English or has no sense of humor, you get a laugh and begin your relationship on a friendly light-hearted note.

Don't use the same greetings with all of your patients every time you see them. Sometimes you can just say, "That's great," when they say they are fine, or "We're here to get you better," if they tell you they are terrible. You can even make small talk: "It sure is a lovely day. What are we doing in a place like this with the sun shining so brightly?"

There are an unlimited number of responses you can use to provide comedic variation. The object is to show that you have a sense of humor and some personality, even if you don't. It's not so hard to practice greetings and see which ones work. After trial and error, you should come off as friendly and witty to most of your patients. Practice these greetings and you are on your way to having great bedside manner.

TREATMENT HUMOR

Practitioners who perform procedures that are either boring or frightening to most patients should find treatment humor extremely helpful. This material doesn't work for simple exams or treating patients under general anesthesia.

When explaining your procedure to a patient, you can get a good laugh or at least set the tone away from seriousness with this offering:

DOCTOR
"During this procedure there will be *absolute-*
ly no pain (pause) for me and my staff."

You emphasize *absolutely*. This line provides a great use of the unexpected to engender comedic relief.

Never pass up an opportunity to make your patients laugh. When your stomach starts talking in the middle of treatment, it can be rather embarrassing if you don't embrace the moment:

DOCTOR
"I guess you realize that's my stomach talking to you.
Please ignore him when he tells you I'm a jerk. I miss
one meal and he carries on like I never feed him."

This little banter turns an embarrassing situation into a light-hearted opportunity to make your patient laugh.

Compliment Humor During Treatment

During the course of treatment, you should compliment the patient often. Terms to use should vary: "You are doing great (so well, fabulous, awesome, fantastic)." At one point immediately after you have given one of these compliments, you say very seriously,

DOCTOR
"I know it's not polite to compliment myself this way."

The patient will usually laugh and you respond:

DOCTOR
"Oh.... I guess you thought I was talking about you all this time."

They will laugh.
Other variations on the compliment humor:

DOCTOR
"You're the best patient I've seen today."

Pause:
"Of course, no one else showed up yet."

Variation:

DOCTOR
"I don't think I have ever seen a patient as good as you."

Pause:
"Of course, considering I'm not the doctor, I guess that's expected."

They laugh. If they jump up from the table, you better go back to the "just kidding" line, but don't worry, most patients get it. You continue:

DOCTOR
"Actually, I'm the maintenance guy and I've seen the doctor doing this hundreds of times while I'm taking out the trash.
You have nothing to worry about."

Variation on the above:

DOCTOR
"I don't think I have ever seen a patient as good as you... at least not since I got my medical license revoked."

Wait for the reaction (a laugh or a look of surprise), and then continue:

DOCTOR
"Don't worry; I should be getting it back any day now. At least that's what my parole officer told me last week. I can't believe they make such a big deal over a few minor felony charges."

A variation using a bragging premise also works well. In the middle of a procedure, you can say:

DOCTOR
"I'd probably be the best dermatologist in the world... if they didn't take away my license. You know, the people at the licensing board in this state seem to take felony charges just a little bit too seriously. I mean what are three or four felonies anyway?
It's not like I robbed a bank.... this year."

These lines usually get such a great response that, on occasion, you may have to halt treatment to let the patient regain their composure.

It takes practice and a little timing to realize a properly placed pause enhances the comedic effect. You may not get a great response every time, but there is nothing more satisfying than making a patient laugh during an intimidating procedure. They will love you and be forever grateful.

Another variation on complimenting patients involves the surprise of insincerity:

DOCTOR
"You are the best patient I've seen today."
You look at your assistant and continue:

DOCTOR
"Mary, did the last patient leave yet?"
She will acknowledge that the last patient left.

DOCTOR
"I really have to be careful. I just told my last patient they were the best patient I saw today. Don't you worry. I won't tell the next patient that....
until I'm sure you've left.

You can try this for a fast line during your treatment:

DOCTOR
"You are the best patient in the chair at the moment."

Pause:
"Okay, you don't think that's much of a compliment, but
I could have said you were the worst patient in the chair
and that would be true, too. Hey, I'm on your side."

There are a hundred ways to compliment your patients with humor, and while they aren't always belly busters, they convey your
personable nature.

DOCTOR
"You are doing so well that I think you are going to win the
patient of the day award."

Pause while they chuckle.

DOCTOR
"I want you to stay by your phone tonight. We make the announcement around four in the morning, and I am almost positive you are going to be the winner."

With a patient you've seen before and whom you have previously
complimented you may continue the theme:

DOCTOR
"You are doing so well, I'm going to put *another* star on your chart."

Pause:
"You have so many stars already; I have nowhere to write
what we are doing today."

The Toy Box For Adults

When the patient is doing well and you want another joke regarding praise, you can use the toy box lines:

DOCTOR
"You are doing so well that I'm going to let you
pick something from our invisible toy box."

They should laugh with your pause.

DOCTOR
"That's right, I'm going to have Mary take you up front and you can
pick out anything you want; a new car, a world cruise, just about
anything you can imagine. I must, however, caution you; Mary will
be watching to make sure you don't try to take more than one prize.
We keep a strict inventory and we'd hate to embarrass you by making you put back any extras you try to sneak out of the office."

The lines offered in this text usually work well with little or no modification depending upon your type of practice. Start slowly and use material that requires one or two easy-to-remember lines. Once you have the confidence that you can get good results, try the longer routines.

LONGER ROUTINES

During the course of treatment, mind reading routines work well:

DOCTOR
"I know what you're thinking."

Pause:
"Your life had little or no meaning until *root canal therapy* with me."

Substitute your procedure the one above: *corn removal, physical therapy, splinter removal, suturing* in the ER, you name it – except heed caution using this line during a proctologic or GYN exam. The patient will laugh, chuckle, grin, or moan. You can stop there if you really need to concentrate on your operation, but if you do the same thing a hundred times every day, you can proceed:

DOCTOR
"Pretty good, huh? You didn't know I could read minds. As a matter of fact, the doctors who studied me at the institute had doubts, too. They told me it wasn't mind reading. They said I was hearing voices."

Pause:
"Can you imagine that? So they insisted that I try this medication. Now you're not going to believe this, but after a few days on the medicine, I couldn't read minds. What a bummer. I was so lonely, that I stopped taking the medicine, and wow, I can read minds again."

Pause for the finale.

DOCTOR
"I know what you're thinking."

Pause:
"And I am not full of..."

Pause:
"I couldn't make out that last word."

A variation on the mind reading goes like this:

DOCTOR
"I know what you're thinking."

Pause:
"You never had this much fun in your life."

You either get the groan, a "not really," or they may even agree, albeit with sarcasm. Look at your assistant and continue:

DOCTOR
"Jill, will you call the company and tell them I want to re-turn the mind reading course immediately?"

Pause:
"No, wait! I think I got it this time."

You look back in the patient's eyes and state:

DOCTOR
"You wish I'd shut up and get done."

Now the patient laughs.

Pause:
"I knew it. In mind reading, those two phrases sound very much alike. Jill you can forget returning the course. I'm just now getting the knack of this mind reading stuff."

If you work on that routine, you will have many happy, loyal pa-tients who will never forget the experience.

Here's a great routine to offer while working on a patient who comes to you in pain or who may expect to have postoperative pain after you complete the procedure.

DOCTOR
"You're going to feel like a new woman."
You wait a moment for it to sink in.

DOCTOR
"Of course I don't want you to get too excited, because
this woman is homeless and sleeps on a park bench."

They laugh and you continue:

DOCTOR
"I guess now you realize you should have been happy with the
woman you were, instead of wanting to feel like a new woman."

Don't rush it; pause and continue:

DOCTOR
"Of course, there's a bright side to everything. This woman you're
going to feel like: she has all her worldly goods in a shoebox."

Pause for the laugh.

DOCTOR
"She never has to worry about closet space."

A few minutes later, a variation works well as it utilizes unexpected irony:

DOCTOR
"You're going to feel like a new woman."

You pause letting them think you forgot you just used that line.

DOCTOR
"You think I forgot that I already told you that, but I didn't."

Pause:
"I just changed my mind. This new woman you're going to feel like...
...she recently left home to join the circus."

As trite as these routines sound, they work almost every time. Once you have mastered this little foray into standup, you will win over just about every patient you see, except for those who are going to report you to the state medical board. Some people just can't take a joke!

TEAM COMEDY

Having a great assistant with a sense of humor helps enormously. If you tell a joke and no one laughs, it takes its toll on your ego and could discourage you from continuing your quest for the perfect bedside manner. Having an assistant who will laugh over and over at the same joke makes your routines appear funny. When your assistant laughs, it lets the patient know you are joking, it tells them they can laugh, and it sets the stage for contagious laughter. Of course you may have to bribe your assistant with a big raise or bonus.

The assistant should be used as the *straight guy* and avoid upstaging the doctor. I once had an assistant who liked my jokes so much she decided to use them before I came into the room. I finally figured it out. After using a surefire winning line, the patient said, "That's funny, but your assistant said the same thing right before you came in." You may have noticed, I said I *once* had an assistant who used my jokes before I came into the room.

Your assistant can be used as the brunt of some of your jokes– but it must be in good fun and never to demean, as that would be inappropriate, and it may ruin your reputation and bedside manner. From the legal perspective, using an employee as the target of repeated jokes can result in a harassment or discrimination suit. You must make sure your assistants aren't offended by your jokes. They usually welcome the humor, as it injects a little appreciated fun into the workplace, but make sure to ask.

Tell the patient how good your assistant is while ending the compliment with a punch line:

DOCTOR
"Jennifer is the best assistant I ever had."

Pause:
"And to think, she couldn't speak English just last week."

The patient and Jennifer will laugh. You pause.

DOCTOR
"I've always liked working with migrant farm work-
ers. I met Jennifer during a grape boycott."

Variation:

DOCTOR
"Jennifer is the best assistant I ever had. You can find some really good help at the home for the criminally insane."

They laugh; you pause and finish with the finale.

DOCTOR
"I met her there when we were roommates."
If your assistant drops an instrument, it of-
fers an opportunity for a line:

DOCTOR
"Mary used to be a knife thrower at the circus. I guess
you can figure out why she's working here with me now.
It's not that she was fired; they just couldn't find anyone to stand there with an apple on their head."

Here's another great series of jokes involving the assistant. While
doing a procedure with your assistant say:

DOCTOR

"Sometimes people take things too literally. Why, just the other day, Mary asked if I needed a certain instrument. I said, 'No, you can hold up.' Now you're not going to believe this, but when I said 'hold up,' she pulled out a gun and took my money and the patient's insurance co-payment."

Stories like this are so unexpected, especially coming from a doctor that they take the patient by surprise. They love the stories and they will love you too.

You follow up with:

DOCTOR

"That was nothing. I was working on a patient the other day and they felt a little discomfort. Being just about done, I said, 'Bare with me.' All of a sudden, I turn around and Mary is standing there naked. I was so embarrassed."

NEEDLE HUMOR

Needle jokes are helpful if you administer injections and want to ease the process. They are a real boost for bedside manner. Needle jokes show a patient you care about them by trying to lighten the experience. By having needle jokes, you combine the elements of humor and compassion in one package.

You should do everything you can to make sure you give a great injection. There is nothing more powerful than giving a painless needle to make a patient love you forever. Usually, some form of distraction including elements of tissue manipulation and talking gets the job done. While topical anesthetics have limited effectiveness, using them helps allay fears and may provide a placebo effect.

When giving a mandibular block injection, or any of the many infiltrations used in dentistry, manipulate the mucosa vigorously with a finger or thumb and pull the mucosa onto the needle in such a manner that the patient very often won't know when the actual injection takes place. This massage technique can distract a patient from most needles and make the experience more pleasant. Assuming you give a great needle, or at least that you are injecting one of the many patients who take injections stoically, there are a number of humorous lines that can enhance your bedside manner.

During or after injecting the star patient:

DOCTOR
"You're doing so well. If I didn't know better, I'd think you were Superman (Superwoman, Superboy, or Supergirl)."

Quite often the patient will chuckle, but don't always expect it. Some stoic patients are concentrating so hard that they may not respond. That doesn't mean they don't appreciate your humor. Continue:

DOCTOR
"You know there's a way to test this theory. I have Kryptonite in the back office and I can use that if necessary."

This often gets the stoic to chuckle.

Variation:

DOCTOR
"I can't believe how good you are at this. Why, just the other day I was treating Superman, and he didn't do as well as you."

Pause:
"Of course, I put Kryptonite in his Novocain
(flu shot, steroid injection)."

Or try this version while injecting:

DOCTOR
"You are doing so well. I can't believe it. Why, just last week, I treated Superman, and you're not going to believe this (pause) he cried. That's right, you're doing better than Superman."
While young boys love that one, most adults laugh at every one of these Superman lines.

While injecting a stoic patient, you can try:

DOCTOR
"I can't believe how good you are at this. You are a rock! I bet your friends call you Rocky."

Pause:
"But it's probably because you can't walk a straight line."

Most patients are not fond of needles–even the stoics. You can use these lines with the patients who make noise and aren't that great since conversation helps get their minds off the experience.
Another good line while injecting uses the addict theme:

DOCTOR
"You are doing so well. If I didn't know better, I'd think you're a B12 addict. Be honest, you just came here to get more B12."

These lines work with allergy shots, flu shots, Novocain, steroid injections into joints, and just about any type of needle you may have to give.
When you get good at using humor with your patients, you will have some of them laughing quite a bit during the course of treatment. You can play upon this by saying things that really get them rolling:

DOCTOR
"I want you to know that your secret is safe with me."

Pause:
"I'm not going to tell the authorities you were laughing
like this during root canal therapy (substitute your procedure here). But I can't be responsible for anything you
tell your friends and loved ones. You tell them how you
were laughing and they may just have you committed."

GOODBYE HUMOR

After a visit you want to leave the patient with a last memento of
your comical style. Depending upon when they need to see you again,
you can use various lines. If you need to see the patient in a few days
or weeks:

DOCTOR
"I'll need to see you in two weeks for another treatment. Now, make sure you don't go around telling all your
friends and family how much you like coming here, or
they'll have you committed (locked up, sent away)."

Or you can try:

DOCTOR
"I know you'll be counting the days in anticipation of another fun
experience. Just don't tell your friends how great this is, or I'll get
so busy I won't be able to see you when you need my services."

If you don't need to see the patient again:

DOCTOR
"Well, I guess it's time to say goodbye. I'm glad we were able
to help you and if you're lucky, you'll never have to see me
again. But we'll be ready for you if you decide you miss us."

Now isn't that better than saying "Have a nice day"?

MEDICAL DEVICES AND HUMOR

An E.R. nurse was examining an elderly woman who happened to be hard of hearing. She put the stethoscope to her chest and said, "Big breaths." The woman replied, "Yes, and they used to be bigger."

Every area of health care has procedures and equipment that naturally invite comedy. Several examples will provide ideas for creating your own lines for equipment you use. Remember, patients love funny doctors, they tell their friends and family to use them, and they will be reluctant to sue warm, compassionate, humorous health-care providers–even if things go wrong.

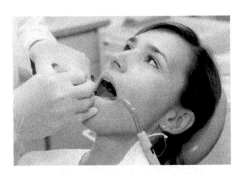

Figure 1: Saliva Ejector

The Saliva Ejector

Most dental procedures begin with the placement of the saliva ejector. This offers a brief comedic opportunity.

DOCTOR
"I'm sure you've seen the saliva ejector. This helps to keep your mouth dry. If it's uncomfortable here, you can put it where you'd like it. Of course, my last patient put it in *my* mouth."

Pause:
"There are some very hostile people out there.
I sure hope you aren't one of them."

Unless your patient is scared out of their wits, they always laugh, and it sets the stage for the rest of the treatment.

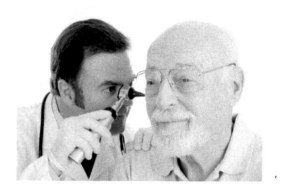

Figure 2: The Otoscopic Exam

The Scope

Many doctors make use of various types of scopes. These devices are used to look inside the nose, ears, throat and just about any accessible cavity. In examining the deep recesses of the throat, an endoscope is inserted into the nose and down the throat. Most often this is done without sedation, and while it doesn't usually hurt, it's rather unpleasant. Less invasive, routine examinations of the ears and nose are done with the otoscope (figure 2). These procedures provide for a moment of humor. After preparing the patient with an explanation of what to expect and just before insertion:

DOCTOR
"After I have a look around in here, I'll let you know if I see anything interesting. The other day I found a pistachio nut, two marbles and a paper clip."

Pause:
"While none of that's true, it makes for an interesting story."

This kind of banter provides an opportunity to relax the patient in an otherwise serious setting.

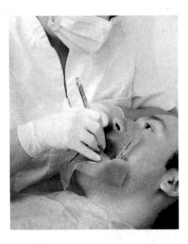

Figure 3: Rubber Dam

The Rubber Dam

In dentistry there is a device called a rubber dam (Figure 3). It's a latex rubber cover that goes over the tooth being treated, and it looks like the patient is wearing a mask. They come in many colors, though green is used by many dentists. While wearing the rubber dam, the patient can't talk back, but they can, most certainly, laugh.

Before placing the rubber dam, explain that you have to put a cover over their tooth to keep germs out of their tooth and dust from getting into their mouth. Once the rubber dam is in place:

DOCTOR
"If you're good today, I'll let you wear this home."

They almost always laugh. In which case, you can continue:

DOCTOR
"This is your color. It looks great on you. Maybe you should consider some green rubber clothing for your fall wardrobe."

Variation:
"I know this sounds kind of odd, but it looks, to me, like you
have a large lettuce leaf growing out of your tooth."

These lines sound lame, but they really work.

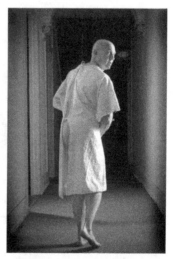

Figure 4: Patient Gown

<u>The Patient Gown</u>

Fashion humor works well with the lovely gowns (figure 4) patients get to wear in the hospital or while being examined in your
office.

When the gynecologist walks into the room with the patient
draped in a flimsy covering, that's a great time to comment:

DOCTOR
"Mary, that sheet looks so good on you.
If you want to wear it home, just let me know."

A similar line works great for the doctor making rounds in the hospital. As you uncover the patient to perform your exam you say:

DOCTOR
"If you're interested, I can get you this same gown with the fur collar."

Variation:

DOCTOR
"I know the people in wardrobe, and if you are interested I can get them to let you wear this gown home."

These comments will make your patients smile and more likely laugh, but more importantly, you will ease their anxiety.

Variation:
Sam is waiting for the digital rectal exam:

DOCTOR
"Sam, that gown looks great on you. It reminds me of the other night when there was a full moon."

Variation:

DOCTOR
"Sam, that gown looks great on you, but if you're planning on going out formal this evening, you might want to try something in a darker shade."

Variation:
"Sam, that gown looks great on you, but before you leave, you might want to consider something to cover your butt."

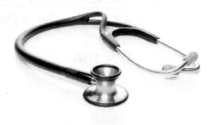

Figure 5: The Stethoscope

<u>*The Stethoscope*</u>

The stethoscope (figure 5) always offers a great way to get a laugh:

DOCTOR
"I know this may be a bit cold, but it's so much better than last month, when I used popsicles to check hearts."

Start rubbing the stethoscope in your hands to warm it up and try this:

DOCTOR
I've had this one out of the freezer for almost two whole minutes. It should be just fine.

<u>HOLIDAY HUMOR</u>

Holidays offer special opportunities to joke with your patients. If you use a green rubber dam, the week of Saint Patrick's Day allows you to joke:

DOCTOR
"What luck! Being that Saint Patrick's Day is just around the corner, I'm going to let you wear this home."

Pause:
"You can tell your friends it's a shamrock put on your tooth
by a lucky leprechaun."

For the entire week after the holiday vary the line:

DOCTOR
"It's a shame you missed our Saint Patrick's Day special. I let all my
patients wear this thing home so they could celebrate in style."

Halloween is another chance for joking with the rubber dam

DOCTOR
"If you're good I'll let you wear this home for trick-or-treat."

Or the variation:

DOCTOR
"It's a shame you missed our Halloween special. I let
all my patients wear this home for trick-or-treat."

The clinic gown works well for the Halloween humor:

DOCTOR
"George, if you'd like, you can wear this gown for Halloween next
week. It makes a great ghost costume if you just cover your butt."

SMOKING HUMOR

Electro-surgery, laser treatments, melting filling material or any
procedure that produces smoke the patient can see or smell offers a
great opportunity to alleviate the patient's fear by using humor:

DOCTOR
"I'm using the laser to remove your wart,
and I don't want you to worry
if you see smoke."

Pause:
"If you hear sirens, that's something you should worry about."

Variation after the pause:

DOCTOR
"If you see men running into the room wearing funny hats and
carrying a big hose, then you have something to worry about."

Another variation after the pause:

DOCTOR
"If you see me and Mary running out of the room yelling things
like 'call 911,' that's something you should worry about."

Another variation after the pause:

DOCTOR
"If you notice a warm feeling in your socks and see smoke
coming out of your shoes, you should let me know."

RIDE IN THE CHAIR HUMOR

Any practice that has a chair or table that tilts backwards lends
to humor:

DOCTOR
"This ride is the best part of the treatment, so I do hope you are
enjoying yourself."

THE LEAD SHIELD

The lead shield offers a cute line if the patient is supine when you place it:

DOCTOR
"If I pull this shield over your head, it means something didn't go as planned. And you really know things didn't go right if you notice the coroner pull up."

Pause:
"But please, don't worry. That almost never happens."

Look at your assistant and continue:

"What do you think, Angie, once or twice a day?"

THE COMMUNICATION COMPASSION COMEDY CONNECTION

As bedrocks of bedside manner, communication, compassion and comedy are often combined to produce a winning formula. Warnings *communicated* in a *comical* manner show you have *compassion* for the patient's wellbeing.

Humor Used To Forewarn Untoward Incidences

It's important to forewarn the patient of possible occurrences that may appear as accidents in order to prevent them from assuming the worst. Every time you place a device that has the potential to come off unexpectedly, or when a snap, crackle, or pop will or could be heard, use a line to forewarn.

In dentistry, the rubber dam can jump off the tooth and frighten the patient. Without explanation or warning it could make the patient think something broke.

DOCTOR:
"Sometimes this can pop off of your tooth. Don't
let it scare you if that happens."

Pause:
"Of course, if it hits me in the head, you'll hear me scream,
and I'll fall to the floor; then you can be scared."

By adding humor to a serious discussion, it helps to allay patient fears.

Another example:

DOCTOR
"When I use the laser to remove your mole, it makes a
popping sound. Don't let the noise frighten you."

Pause:
"Of course, if you hear a loud popping sound and I fall to the floor,
it's probably a sniper unhappy about the last mole I removed."

Before the necessity of complicated informed consents that list every possible risk of treatment, many oral surgeons got involved in situations requiring them to pay for costly dental care after a tooth adjacent to the one they pulled broke. Patients would often blame the surgeon for the accident even knowing that the adjacent teeth were ready to crumble. Since patients may sign informed consents without reading or understanding them, it is best to forewarn of potential risks in a humorous fashion to prevent legal entanglement.

DOCTOR
"Whenever we pull a tooth, there is the possibility that the tooth
next to the one we pull can break and need involved treatment to
save it, or sometimes it also needs to be pulled. It's not too likely
to happen, but unfortunately that is a risk of pulling any tooth."

Pause:
"Of course now that I have this new plastic explosive
I use to remove teeth, it almost never happens."
If the patient doesn't laugh, add:
"I'm just kidding."

When delving in to the world of comedy, go slowly. Try one or two lines that are easy to remember and practice them until it becomes second nature. Once you get the hang of jesting and have the confidence that you really can be funny, go for the longer lines. Develop ways to keep track of what lines you use so that you avoid looking like you use the same lines over and over. While you can't remember every line you used with every patient, you can have first visit lines, second visit lines, lines to greet first time patients, and so forth. This will keep you from looking scripted. While bedside manner is a compilation of many traits, the power of humor is very close to the top.

THE BUSINESS OF MEDICINE

---

*"But doctor, you pulled the wrong tooth. You pulled a
perfectly good tooth for nothing."*

"No I didn't. I'm going to charge you for it."

Profit should not be the prime motivator in the health-care professions, however, there is nothing wrong with selling medicine as long as the health and welfare of the patient is placed above all else. While we think of the plastic surgeon or the cosmetic dentist as the salesmen of the health-care industry, every doctor is really selling something to someone as ignoble as that sounds. Even the oncologist and cancer surgeon are selling their particular protocol and service. After all, who doesn't go for the second opinion? Most patients don't understand the medicine, even after you explain it well. What they do understand are the components of bedside manner. If you are the doctor with the great bedside manner, they come back to you. When you have it, you've essentially sold them on you as much as, if not more than, the protocol.

Once the student graduates from one professional school or another, they are exposed to an onslaught of programs and lectures explaining how to make more money, spend less time in the office, and do better quality service. The problem with these promises is that the only one accomplishing these noble goals is the person on the lecture circuit who is spending less time in the office, making a lot of money from all the attendees, and providing better quality in that they are not in the office performing iatrogenics.

The big business of medicine is not all bad. Wherever there is a lot of money, innovation and technology flourish. Once dentists realized that they could sell cosmetics and advertise the procedures, money poured into new materials that never might have been developed without the promise of big profits.

In medicine, there are many technologies that may have never come to pass, and new and exciting drugs could never be developed without the extensive research dollars generated by the pharmaceutical companies. The promise of vast riches will make an artificial heart and the cure of cancer realities.

When you develop your selling philosophies and protocols for elective treatment, it is imperative to make sure you are not pushing unnecessary procedures, or procedures your patients cannot afford. There are many lecturers out there telling you how to help patients find the money for procedures that you convince them they need. You have to ask yourself if they need the service or if you are just pushing it past many other things they may now have to do without because you sold them a bill of goods.

Finding patients easy credit for elective procedures may put them in debt for years. You have to be a compassionate practitioner and make sure you aren't part of the vehicle that takes the patient to bankruptcy.

Before advertising in the health-care professions, patients and doctors had a different mindset. Patients came in when they had a problem and doctors addressed the problem. Prevention and lifestyle was encouraged, but there was little, if any, selling. Now gurus teach you how to advertise effectively, literally chart monthly production, increase sales of the most lucrative procedures, offer financing for better case acceptance, and encourage staff to sell in order to participate in production goals that have to continually go up. This sounds a lot more like corporate America than the medical profession.

You have to ask yourself what distinguishes you as a professional. Patients aren't stupid. They can often see through all the hype and recognize a pitchman. Your credibility rapidly fades when the patient perceives you as a salesman. It's imperative to learn that a big part of being compassionate is not selling your patients things they don't need and can't afford.

We have gone from an era where doctors weren't allowed to make claims of superiority to daily advertising that makes claims, direct or implied, that one hospital and their doctors are better than all others. How does that make a patient feel if he just had a prostate operation at one hospital and hears that another hospital has the best technique and way of treating his problem? Maybe it's time to rethink professionalism.

MALPRACTICE CLAIMS

Two kids were trying to figure out what game to play.
One suggested, "Let's play doctor."
"Good idea." said the other. "You operate, and I'll sue."

A Philadelphia OBGYN: "I never thought it would
come to this. I no longer have a private practice. I
had to sell out to the hospital once the malpractice
insurance premiums got too expensive. Now they
have midwives doing the deliveries, and I only come
in for complications. They know they are going to
get sued for just about everything that goes wrong,
so they go with the flow and reduced costs with the
midwives. The obstetricians are leaving this town left
and right, and they are relocating to friendlier cities."

Since many malpractice cases are not based on medical mistakes, even the best doctors can, and most likely will, get sued. The doctors with the best bedside manner, who learn to practice defensively, are the ones less likely to end up in court.

A TALE OF TWO DOCTORS

Doctor 1 – One surgeon did a routine I&D (incision and drainage) on a patient who presented with some numbness in the surrounding tissues. After the procedure, the patient sued the surgeon claiming the numbness was caused by the I&D. This particular doctor acts pleasant to his patients, but utilizes none of the skills associated with bedside manner. He doesn't exhibit any compassion or humor and his communication skills are lacking. He explains options, risks, and consequences minimally. During treatment he makes no effort to interact with the patients. The patient was successful in winning the case on a settlement as the insurance company told the doctor they couldn't mount any type of defense due to his lack of informed consent.

Doctor 2 – This radiologist experienced the misfortune of having a fifty-pound x-ray unit fall off the wall mount onto a patient causing a corneal injury. Fortunately, it was a glancing blow and didn't do extensive damage. The doctor, skilled in all aspects of bedside manner, had formed an immediate bond with this first-time patient before the accident. The night of the accident he made a trip to the patient's home and sat with her and her husband to tell them how sorry he was for her injury. The patient returned to this doctor for follow-up treatment and she told him how all of her friends and family told her she should sue him. She further explained how she liked him so much and that the visit to her home precluded any chance of her taking any legal action.

Patients sue for the most unforeseen reasons, quite often due to financial considerations, unexpected outcomes, and sometimes because there are personality conflicts. Naturally, claims have to have merit or they will be dismissed, but that doesn't mean patients can't institute legal action. Once you go through the nightmarish process of a lawsuit, you will understand why it is better to have patients that love you. They will almost never want to sue you, even when things go wrong.

Some doctors believe patients come to them solely for their expertise. Of course they come for their expertise, but they would actually like to have a friendly doctor who explains things to them and shows some compassion. So, like it or not, you may have to make some major adjustments to the way you greet and treat your patients. Yes, you are going to have to say good morning with a smile on your face. It's a good beginning.

The February 19, 1997, issue of the JAMA offers a better understanding of the way bedside manner can help reduce lawsuits. Specific conversational behaviors were noted in doctors who were never sued compared to those with a history of malpractice claims.

The manner in which doctors spoke with patients was a big factor in the way they were perceived. The tone of voice, explaining what the patient could expect and making sure the patient understood information or instructions, helped. It was also found that primary care physicians who used humor were less likely to be sued.

Physicians who had not been sued also spent more time with their patients (18.3 versus 15 minutes). Having patients talk about their concerns and express their opinions went a long way toward connecting with doctors in a positive manner.

Patients don't want to be rushed, ignored, or treated rudely. It is imperative to take time to answer patients' questions, especially when things may have not gone well. It never fails; the patient with complications shows up in the middle of a hectic day. While the tendency is to rush the patient, this is the time to pay special attention to their needs. Make sure you explain what went wrong and when you are done ask if they have any questions. If they interrupt in the middle of your explanation, you can politely say, "I want to answer all of you questions as soon as I've finished explaining things to you."

THE INFORMED CONSENT

The informed consent is a matter of professional necessity and offers the best way to communicate with your patients in a manner that helps prevent lawsuits and defend against them if you end up in court. A common problem with informed consents that leads to the courtroom relates to making light of, or neglecting to mention, the potential for complications. When there is a good chance the patient will miss several weeks of work after a procedure, you have an obligation to mention the possibility to the patient. Most everyone I know would be rather perturbed to have an unexpectedly long recovery. It always pays to make the prediction for more difficulty than less.

It is common for doctors to downplay expected postoperative sequelae in order to sell the case. I suspect there are many people out there who might reconsider elective plastic surgery if they knew how difficult some of the healing might actually be for them.

It is your job to educate the patient and give them a realistic understanding of the procedures. Explain things clearly and use terms that are understandable. Try to present your explanations with the proper balance between what is expected and what could go wrong. You must warn the patient about the very worst-case scenario without scaring them away from the preferred treatment:

- Begin by explaining that the procedure is not usually a worrisome event if that is the case.
- With risky procedures that have many problems associated with them, be forthright.
- Explain any and all adverse possibilities that could occur. Even if the occurrence is one in a thousand, the complication is one hundred percent when it happens to your patient.

Here is an example of a thorough explanation with an element of humor. It can help you formulate a script for all of the procedures you perform:

DOCTOR
"Root canal therapy is not usually a big deal. As a matter of fact most of my patients tell me it's the greatest thing they ever experienced."

Pause:
The patient will usually smile, laugh, or make comment. You smile back and continue.

DOCTOR
"Of course I'm just kidding. The reality is that you could have some
discomfort or pain afterward and this is completely normal. A small
percent of the cases could experience pain for a few days. It's usually handled well with some Tylenol or Advil and it settles down.
In rare cases you could have a flare-up, whereby you have pain
and swelling that could get so bad you'd want the tooth pulled.
This is rare and almost never happens."

If this patient has a severe flare-up, they have been forewarned
and are less likely to assume the practitioner did something wrong.

No matter what procedures you perform, whether orthopedics,
cosmetics, general surgery or whatever, structure your consent so
that it describes worst case scenarios. While you don't want to fright-
en your patient, it is only fair to let them know of possible consequences. You must always offer disclaimers stating that these things
rarely happen, but you are trying to let them know all possibilities.

I saw a young male patient for a postoperative complication of
pain and swelling. As soon as I entered the room, the mother was on
attack mode. "In all my experience with root canals, I never saw anything like this," she asserted. I asked her, "How much is all your experience?" She told me that she had two root canals. I almost laughed,
but refrained, knowing that great bedside manner dictates holding
back laughter in situations like this one. I just let a friendly smile
show as I bit hard onto my tongue. "It's interesting that in all your
experience you may not have seen anything like this, but I've treated
around a thousand cases each year for the past thirty years, and I've
seen this a few times." She didn't seem to care in the least that I may
have had more experience than her.

I looked into my notes and saw the specific entry warning the
possibility of a flare-up notated because this particular case was the
type that has an increased chance of complications. I looked up from

the chart and said, "Mrs. Smith, I see a note here that indicates we discussed the possibility that this tooth could flare-up. Do you remember that discussion?" She went on to apologize for attacking me, and I told her I'm sure I'd react the same way (you have to lie sometimes). I, again, explained how the dormant infection could act up, that the antibiotic wasn't doing the trick, that we would increase the dose, and, if necessary, switch to something stronger. I took all the time necessary to explain and answer the mother's questions while knowing the next patient was probably getting annoyed waiting for me as I went further behind schedule. That's bedside manner. That's avoiding lawsuits when things go wrong.

Even the best-loved doctor may get sued if the damages are large enough. A death after a routine procedure will surely see some legal discovery to determine if the doctor could be at fault. By arming yourself with all the proper documentation, and by being there for the patient and family in times of trouble, you provide the comfort your patients deserve, and keep yourself safe.

NO SKILL REQUIRED PERSONALIZED SERVICE

"Doctor, I'd rather have a baby than this root canal."

"That's fine with me, just make up your mind
so I know which way to tilt the chair."

Not everyone can have a stellar personality that encompasses all the facets of great bedside manner. Even without highly advanced social skills there are four things you can do to give a perception of good bedside manner. They are relatively easy to implement, they make patients feel important, and show that you care about them as people.

1. Follow-up Phone Calls

Calling *every* patient the night after their procedure is one of the most highly regarded expressions of bedside manner, as well as being an effective practice booster. This small act exemplifies concern and compassion for the patient's wellbeing. Of course, this isn't necessary after a simple examination, but after any significant procedure, a follow-up call from the doctor to ask how the patient is doing goes a long way to cement a lasting relationship. Something as simple as the removal of a mole, to the more invasive outpatient surgeries, offer great opportunities to see how the patient is feeling. Patients appreciate the concern and care expressed and late-night emergency calls are often eliminated since postoperative issues can be discussed at this time.

When you refer a patient to a specialist, you should call the patient after they have had their visit. By asking how things went and what they thought of the specialist, you show that you care. The conversation doesn't have to be lengthy; you can get the job done in just a few minutes. Your patients will begin to think of you as a friend and appreciate that you're accessible. Most doctors are busy enough and they don't want to take the time to go that extra mile, but if you find the time to make that special call, you will stand out among your peers. It doesn't involve learning any new skills and there is no personality requirement to be thoughtful. If you can't find it in your personality, temperament, or schedule to make the calls, at least have someone from your office make the calls for you – but nothing compares to the personal touch. Find the time.

2. Refreshments

Offering tea or coffee with some light refreshments in the waiting room displays an overall feeling of kindness and generosity, while not requiring much on your part. Patients interpret a comfortable office ambiance that makes them feel good as a positive connection to the doctor.

3. Correspondence

Personal letters at holiday time and on each patient's birthday are great ways to show you care. If computer generated letters and cards are used, make sure they look like personalized correspondence. Hand-address each envelope and use a postage stamp instead of meter postage.

When holiday letters are sent to a family, make sure only one letter is sent to each family and not each individual in the household. Sending five letters to the same address looks careless. Make sure you scribe a new letter each year so patients don't get the same one, year after year. Remember, you are trying to look like you offer personalized service.

4. Giveaways

Everyone likes giveaways – something for nothing. There's a very popular bank that offers the best service around, and they give away tons of free pens. Customers flock there. Of course it's more than just pens, but this bank understands the power of freebies. The medical and dental suppliers figured that one out long ago. Many professionals buy more products and supplies when they get a "toy." They often prefer to deal with the companies that have the best giveaway programs. As unprofessional as that may sound, it is a true fact of marketing. You can utilize this same method to sell you and your office. All you have to do is offer little gifts and giveaways and you shall have very happy patients who feel good about visiting you.

You may not realize it, but everyone who gives child patients a little toy or a lollypop is already employing this very same technique. Kids can't wait to go back and get that rubber worm, magnifying glass or other assorted treasures that adults don't appreciate. Now all you have to do is offer adult patients an equivalent reward. You don't want to overdo it with free gimmicks at each visit. However, you can have holiday presents you send to good patients. Offer a gadget at especially long or difficult visits and tell the patient it's their reward for making your day go so well by being such a good patient. Everyone likes a compliment and everyone likes something for nothing. You don't have to learn anything new, you can have no personality and you can still win over your patients with little gifts here and there when appropriate.

ADVERSARIAL RELATIONSHIPS

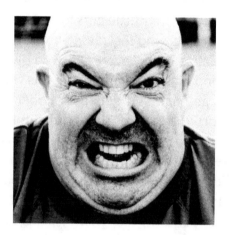

When asked how he deals with the ornery, miserable, nasty patient, a busy urologist relates that he tells them that their case is more involved than what he treats, and that he would like them to see another specialist in town who might be able to better manage their problem. This way he avoids dealing with a patient who would make his life miserable. Directing the misanthropic patient to a teaching hospital or a boutique practice, where they have time to placate the difficult patient, relieves stress and burnout.

While referring the difficult patient to another office solves one problem, it may result in others. The patient could spread the word that you are not good enough to treat complex cases or that you gave up on caring for them. This could adversely affect your reputation and send the wrong message to others keeping them away from your care. It may be best to tell the patient who second guesses you and criticizes your treatment protocol that you feel they would be well served by a doctor who can better manage their concerns. A good script for accomplishing the dismissal of a patient follows in the section on *the nasty patient.*

It is extremely difficult to go through your lifetime of practice without incurring some adversarial relationships. You must avoid or mitigate such incidents to protect your reputation and the integrity of your practice. Doctors with great bedside manner have fewer incidents; however, it is inevitable that even they will not please everyone all the time. Learning how to handle adversarial relationships requires various strategies to defuse situations while maintaining your sanity.

There are several areas of human interaction that are prone to misunderstanding, disagreement, or conflict. Good communication skills are necessary to both avoid and remedy adversarial incidents.

OFFICE POLICY

Rules and policies must be established for an office to run properly. Policy and exceptions must be taught to your staff so you don't have to handle every problem. Your policies should be flexible enough to show compassion without having patients take advantage of your kindness. An office that is too rigid tends to dilute the doctor's efforts at bedside manner.

There are times you have to give in to patient demands, but it should be the exception; and when it causes tension between you and your staff, make sure you explain to them why you gave in and hear their point of view so that you remain attuned to their feelings.

Money Matters

Non-payment of bills or disagreement over fees for services rendered has great potential for adversarial conflict. Strict monetary policy makes matters worse. Many patients leave a practice because of money issues. Exceptions should be made to help a patient who has financial problems, when fees weren't clearly explained, or when insurance companies don't pay what was expected. Certainly, you don't want patients to take advantage of your goodwill, but any financial policy needs to have some flexibility.

If you explain to your staff in advance those situations where payment policy may be changed, you won't be undermining their authority at the front desk. Helping a needy patient through a difficult time may be the best booster for your bedside manner as it personifies compassion. Offering a refund for a failed procedure doesn't have to be construed as an admission of guilt. It can be a wonderful practice booster for the patient who may not have understood the prognosis issues related to their treatment.

Financial policy exceptions need to have limitations. You don't want to become the neighborhood banker. Sadly, some people pay bills that have to be paid and put off payment to the good-hearted doctor who doesn't have any policy about collection of fees.

Scheduling

Coming late to appointments and repeatedly missing appointments leads to adversarial relations when you try to remedy the situation. It is important to identify those patients who are repeat offenders and utilize scheduling remedies noted in the chapter on the waiting room.

Rather than sending a late patient home, it may be best to have them seated and let the doctor do a cursory exam and explain why he needs them to return and be on time so he will be able to accomplish the procedure.

DOCTOR

"We're lucky that today I only had to do a minor procedure. Next visit, I need much more time
so please don't be late for that appointment."

I worked for an office that refused to see patients if they came more than fifteen minutes late. Since each visit was scheduled for thirty minutes, it could be argued that it was reasonable enough to reappoint patients coming that late. While sitting around reading a magazine, waiting for my patient, I heard her arrive and explain to the secretary how she waited in the storm for the bus to come, and it was running late. The secretary proceeded to tell the patient she would have to reschedule. I intervened and told the patient I would see her. Naturally, the secretary wasn't very happy.

Had I let the secretary turn away this old woman, drenched by the storm, I would have validated the poor reputation this office developed over the years. You have to have a heart and not worry so much about going to lunch late. Better yet, in your office, set up policies that prevent adversarial situations.

PATIENT BEHAVIOR

The Dictating Patient

Numerous patient behaviors result in conflict. There are those who like to dictate treatment. The patient can refuse treatment, get other opinions, or not follow directions; but dictating treatment is not permitted. This doesn't mean the doctor shouldn't be open to patient suggestions or ideas they may have garnered in some alternative therapy search. Showing interest in their ideas makes the patient feel validated in spending the time to do the research, while disregarding or mocking their efforts lends toward bad feelings.

You cannot let a patient dictate malpractice. If the patient says they want you to perform a procedure in a manner that you know is malpractice, having them sign a waiver does not remove your liability. A patient refusing x-rays is a common example. A signed waiver doesn't excuse the doctor's responsibility when untoward results occur from not having the proper x-rays.

The Nasty Patient

An experienced psychologist:
"I have been taught never to try to reason with an
angry or irrational patient, it just doesn't work.
What I will use is a 'joining technique' simply try-
ing to join with the patient where he/she is at
with the anger that they have. It shows the patient
that you not only hear what they are saying but
also that you understand what they are feeling."

Truly belligerent patients should be dismissed from your practice. While you may have the temptation to tell this type of patient what you think about them, it is best to show kindness.

"Mr. Smith, I am so sorry that you feel this way about... (your treatment outcome; our office policy; my staff; me etc.). The most important thing needed in a doctor patient relationship is trust and comfort with the doctor. I want you to have the best available treatment to help resolve your problems. With this in mind, I will do everything I can to help you find a doctor who can fulfill all of your needs. I would like to recommend... (Offer the name of another doctor or the name of a hospital based practice.). Let me do some research and get back to you with a recommendation."

If you prefer to avoid making a recommendation, you can refer the patient to the county medical/dental society to help them find a new doctor. Make sure you document all the details of these encounters in the patient chart. Dismissal of any patient should be followed up with a letter to the patient outlining the recommendation and the offer to see them for any emergency needs for the next thirty days (check with your licensing board to see how long you have to offer emergency care to the dismissed patient). This documentation helps defend against accusations of abandonment.

It's difficult, even for the irrational, belligerent patient, to argue with your concern for their wellbeing and effort to find help for them. You can't please the world, and there is no reason you need the added stress of an inconsiderate, nasty patient unless you like the challenge.

Staff will often run back to warn doctors about some terribly obnoxious patient. These patients may be on antidepressants or other psychotropic drugs. They may have some personality disorder that makes them adversarial with most of the people in their lives. Make your staff aware of such personality types and how to recognize them by the nature of the patient's behavior. Another clue may be garnered by reading their medical history and noting the medications they take. Your staff will be better able to deal with the belligerence knowing there is a medical reason for the abhorrent behavior. Quite often patients who act antisocial are bipolar, depressed, or dealing with some such illness. Others may just be miserable, have low tolerance for stress, dealing with family or work problems or they may be inconsiderate of others. Once you and your staff recognize this reality, you will not take affronts personally.

Sometimes You Just Can't Win

A pediatrician was threatened by the mother of his patient. It escalated to such an extent that the police were called, and she was arrested. Eventually, she was convicted on various charges and served time in prison for her terroristic threats. To this day, the doctor is still worried about this woman and the threat she poses to him and his family.

The Let's Make A Deal Patient

Some patients may try to bargain for services. You have the option to make deals, though that may not appear very professional. Hopefully, your fees are based on the value of the services rendered and should not be discounted except for financial hardship or perhaps as a discount for multiple procedures. The best way to handle a bargaining patient is to explain that your fees are the same for everyone and that if you were to offer a discount to one patient you would have to offer it to all patients to be fair. You may want to have senior fees for the elderly who rather often ask if they are available. By offering compassionate answers to patients' requests, you keep your bedside manner intact even if you don't give the patient the answer they desire.

The Nasty Letter

When patients make written complaints against you, your staff, or office policies, it is best to respond personally to their concerns either by phone or by mail. Avoid making incriminating statements that can be used against you in court, but don't be afraid to defend your polices in a professional and respectful manner. If the patient complaint is justified, be willing to apologize for inappropriate policies, staff behavior, or personal behavior. Patients will appreciate the time you take to respond, and many times you can resolve the misunderstanding and retain a patient who becomes loyal and admiring rather than the one who makes negative comments all around town. If you don't have the time or the ability to respond personally, have a highly competent, compassionate staff member take on the responsibility. Always document in the patient chart any response you or your staff makes by phone or by written communication.

STAFF

Some would argue that relations with staff shouldn't affect bedside manner, however, if your staff isn't on your side, they can convey negativity to patients either subconsciously or overtly by making negative comments. Negativity always undermines the doctor-patient relationship by placing doubts as to why others may not like the provider.

Negative behaviors or comments by staff should not be tolerated. Most doctors who have great bedside manner are usually warm and caring to their staff, and the staff is usually very fond of the doctors. This positive relationship is conveyed to the patients either overtly or subtly in the way they show respect. A positive relationship with staff validates the patient's good feelings about the doctor.

You have to be creative in order to please your patients and staff. You need to have them both on your side.

The patient is always right philosophy is a detriment to relationships with staff. No matter what the staff says regarding policy, if the patient complains, and the doctor acquiesces, the staff may become furious, and justifiably so.

In cases where you let the patients have their way, they will love you. However, catering to pushy patients will invariably inconvenience others. There are times when you should dismiss from your practice adversarial patients who can't get along with your staff and abide by your policies. A happy staff is much more important than a few happy dysfunctional patients.

COLLEAGUES

Negative comments about other professionals are not appropriate. While some health-care providers feed upon making negative comments about colleagues to make themselves look superior, it is not professional nor ethical. It does get some patients to assume you must be very good since you recognize the failings of the other provider, but it also undermines the profession making patients believe other doctors are incompetent. Unless you know the circumstances of the other doctor's relationship and treatment encounters with the patient, you cannot comment fairly.

If you find a colleague who invariably provides poor advice or treatment to common patients, you have a duty to contact this provider to make sure your judgment is valid, make recommendations, and if problems continue, consider a report to the medical board.

If a colleague contacts you in an adversarial manner, maintain a professional demeanor, listen to the complaint, and indicate you will respond to the issue after some thought. It would be best to get counsel from other colleagues if the complaint regards treatment protocol. When you get back to the provider, you can have your response and remedy well thought out and organized.

LOYALTY AND THE HMO

The elderly gentleman is about to leave the urologist's office after getting his treatment for impotence. He goes to the secretary and asks her why the fellow who just left was given a prescription for Viagra and he got Popsicle sticks and duct tape. "Oh, that gentleman has fee-for-service insurance and you have the HMO coverage."

One of the most disheartening aspects of bedside manner is how quickly loyalty goes out the window when the patient has to pay a few dollars more for your service than for the provider who belongs to their HMO. It's not hard to understand how patients are willing to leave your practice if the out-of-pocket expense is considerable. After all, for many patients, coming up with hundreds of dollars to pay your bill is motivation enough to switch to a doctor whose bedside manner doesn't compare to yours. When they leave your practice to save a few dollars by using a network provider, you have a right to feel betrayed.

As much as you may wish to think HMO's will not affect you, it can happen. There was a time when doctors believed their patients would never leave them for medical plans that forced them to see foreign practitioners with language barriers and doctors with no bedside manner, but they were sadly mistaken.

Some doctors gravitate toward fields offering cosmetic procedures that today seem immune to managed health care. They may also fall to market forces one day. Already, patients go to other countries to have breast augmentation and other elective procedures. Clinics in most every country offer cosmetic procedures at discounted fees. Foreign doctors can be more competitive because costs are less, and they don't have the regulation and threat of lawsuits found in America.

Remember, many patients assume every practitioner is competent. They think the procedures done at a discount mill are going to be the same as at your office.

You have a few choices when dealing with managed care. You can join every plan on the market and schedule a hundred patients each day, you can strive for the boutique office and limit your practice to those who want to pay your fees, or you can accept managed care plans that allow you to provide decent care without seeing too many patients.

Many young practitioners feel compelled to join every HMO in order to build a practice. That may be your reality, and in time your practice should grow exponentially. But try to avoid the trappings that prevent you from providing exceptional professional care, cause burnout, and never let you develop your full potential toward a great bedside manner. Once you live a lifestyle based on working excessive hours, it can be difficult to give up.

As you find yourself seeing more patients than is reasonable, reassess the benefits of bringing in an associate or of dropping the less fruitful plans, thus allowing you to grow a practice more suited to your personality and desire to live a balanced life. You can't have any semblance of bedside manner, nor can you provide optimal care, if you have to see too many patients.

GERIATRICS

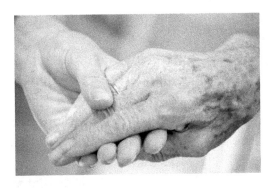

The elderly couple consulted with the young doctor and told him they would like to engage in sex and wanted to make sure they were doing it properly for their age. While it seemed like an odd request, he took them into the examination room and let them go to town. At the completion, he told them they were doing just fine and all should be well. He even congratulated them on such an exceptional performance. The next week, and the week after that they were back in his office making the same request and he let them engage again. Becoming suspicious by the forth week, he asked, "You folks seem to be doing everything just right. Why do you keep coming back here?" "Well, doc," replied the old man, "at the nursing home we have no privacy, and a hotel room is eighty-five dollars. When we come here, our Medicare co-pay is just ten bucks."

Treating the elderly is a special field. These patients need an entirely different approach to care and that's why there are specialists who treat them. However, most everyone sees elderly patients at times. Those of you who master bedside manner will see more than others since your younger patients who would never go anywhere else are going to bring their parents to see you.

The elderly may require more time for you to hear their complaints and for you to explain treatment options. If you are a rushed practitioner you will fail at treating the elderly. They can be a challenge because they may not understand your explanations and they may not be compliant in following treatment protocols and postoperative directions.

The elderly often move, explain, and understand more slowly, resulting in delays that can frustrate you. Something as simple as asking an elderly patient to give you their list of medications can take an inordinate amount of time. Making provisions to get all necessary information before the appointment will help avoid wasted time.

You must be willing to explain everything several times, utilizing simple drawings and written instructions that you will copy for them to take home. It is best to have an elderly patient come to see you with a younger person or a spouse who may help to remember what you tell them and to help them decide upon treatment options. If you see they are confused, you should offer them time to "think it over" and reschedule.

If an elderly patient is in your treatment room alone, always ask if they are with someone. Now is the time to bring back their company, or you will have to explain everything twice when they announce they'd like you to repeat what you just told them to their spouse, sibling, child, or caretaker.

The elderly are often hard of hearing and intolerant of loud music. Consider turning down the volume of your treatment room music so that they can better hear your explanations. If you have the option to play calming music, do so.

You should expect questions that may be repeated several times. Be tolerant and willing to repeat your explanation and speak louder if necessary. But don't start out assuming they can't hear you, as yelling is insulting if their hearing is fine.

Taking a few more moments to clarify things is very much appreciated by the elderly and those accompanying them to see you. Try to project into the future when you may appreciate some kind young practitioner taking the extra time to help you when you are old.

For many older patients the relationship with a doctor is one of the few opportunities they have for conversation and the visit is often enjoyed, especially if you are amiable. Some patients may actually feign complaints to visit with you. It is imperative to keep this in mind when making a diagnosis. If unrecognized, the phenomenon (*doctor visit social time*) can lead to unnecessary tests and treatment.

You never want to discount a patient's complaints, but if you suspect they are using medical excuses to visit with you, have a heart and humor them as best as your time allows. The visit may be the best medicine you could ever prescribe. If they visit frequency or time involved becomes intrusive, you may have to refer the patient for specialty evaluation, telling them you no longer have any solutions for their symptoms.

If you have the time, try to set up ongoing appointments at three-month intervals telling the older patient you want to check on them regularly. This gives them something to look forward to, and the ten minutes you offer is an act of kindness that can make you feel alive.

THE PHYSICAL PLANT

The office environment is a reflection of the health-care provider much in the same manner as is dress and personal grooming. Since bedside manner is the perception patients have regarding your expertise, personality and very being, you can't ignore your environment. Office design is vital to the patient experience. As a general rule, make sure your surroundings won't offend anyone. While you may never please all of the people all of the time, try not to offend any of the people most of the time. Physical plant design techniques that enhance your image are often so subtle your patients may not notice, but they work.

The Private Entrance

If you are the type of practitioner who can't get to the office on time, or if you have emergencies that require you to arrive late, a private entrance is essential. Nothing seems more inconsiderate than a doctor's tardy entry met by a waiting room full of patients.

Treatment Room Privacy

Do whatever you can to keep your office a private enclave. You should isolate patients from each other. You don't want *patient A* to hear your conversations with *patient B*. The last thing you want a patient to hear is another patient in pain. Separate patients as much as possible, by utilizing three treatment rooms. The middle room is used for simple procedures. The two end rooms are used for actual treatment. This provides approximately fifteen feet and two walls of insulation to separate patients undergoing involved treatment. They are unlikely to hear confidential information about the other patient (HIPPA regulations), noise that may frighten them, complaints or financial discussions.

Equipment

Patients like to go to the doctor with the best bedside manner and the best facility. No matter how kind and personable you may be, if there is another practitioner who is just as nice they will pick the one with the latest technological innovations. Patients want the latest and the greatest care from that great doctor. Never cut corners to save money when it comes to your equipment. Be willing to invest in new technologies and learn to master them. Use the best quality materials. There is usually a reason certain items cost more, and in the end, you save money and aggravation by avoiding failing parts and equipment that need to be replaced too often. When that failing part is an implant or device placed in the patient, the consequences of not using the best can be demonstrable.

Some very mediocre doctors have all the modern equipment, and their patients are duly impressed. While the equipment doesn't make the doctor, it certainly helps the image. Don't fool yourself into thinking you never have to embrace new technologies or the level of care you provide will not be at the highest level possible.

Placement of the treatment table or chair should always be facing the entrance of the room. Many design consultants want the patient facing the window when there's a nice view. This positioning puts the patient in a vulnerable state-of-mind. The patient should always see you enter so that you don't startle them from behind, and they should always see the exit. On a subliminal level, the apprehensive patient doesn't want to feel trapped or enclosed.

The Accessible Doctor

Make sure you have phones in each treatment room so you can take calls if necessary. When a patient sees you answer a call to speak with another doctor or patient, they see that you are accessible, but never take personal calls in front of the patient. Phone conversations with friends or business calls are resented. Excuse yourself if you must, and make it look like you have to take a call for professional reasons.

Make sure your staff has nonverbal or cryptic ways to communicate who is on the other line. "Your stockbroker needs to speak with you" is not an announcement that should be made for the patient to hear. Speaking to your stockbroker in front of patients is offensive. Taking personal calls from your spouse or children in front of the patient is another taboo, especially when the patients wait inordinate amounts of time to see you. They want your attention.

After-hours accessibility is a must in most practices. Either a highly efficient *answering service* or a good *answering machine* that calls your cell phone helps a patient reach you when in distress. Occasionally test your system to make sure it works.

A patient wanted to make an appointment with a psychologist: "I called six offices. None of the offices answered the phone. One had an answering service that put me on hold for way too many minutes with static-filled music of an unprofessional genre. When the woman got back to me, she had to look up on a list to see if this was Dr. Smith's office. She had no idea of his hours, his fees or where he was located. Can an answering service be any more impersonal? The answering machine offices were not much better. While I could leave my number for a call back, one machine noted that 'you must speak loud or the device will hang up on you. Sorry for the inconvenience.' Maybe that doctor should consider buying a machine that works! The others offered that I leave my name with no mention of hours, location, or anything about when I could expect a return call. They did all caution that if I was having an emergency I should go to the emergency room. I suppose that protects them when it takes days to return their calls."

Many types of health-care providers, like the psychologists in the above examples, don't have traditional offices or secretaries. The home office is often the venue and taking calls is not offered when they are not in or when they are seeing patients. It may be best to consider a full service answering service that has the ability to make appointments and provide any information that new or existing patients require. The first contact most new patients have before seeing you is whoever answers your phone. Make sure it is a pleasant experience or you may never see many patients.

The Distracted Patient

Some doctors like to keep the patient busy with headphone music because they want to do their work unimpeded by conversation. Some doctors have nothing to say and love to give the patient something to do to mask their lack of personality.

If you have the patient who asks to use headphones, let them. They need the distraction of the music more than they want to hear your witty monologue. If you have nothing to say, or if you make disturbing noises, like drilling, encourage the use of headphones. In either case, make sure the patients know that you are there for them, and if they need anything they should let you know. That thought is comforting.

Decorating

Office décor should be tasteful and play to your patient base. Conservative choices are less likely to offend even if they may not be your personal taste. Avoiding excesses and extremes while employing good taste in decorating will most likely please just about everyone.

Utilizing rich furnishings and decorative accessories makes some patients feel that the provider overcharges them and they are paying for all the amenities. Some practitioners actually think the more costly the office looks the better their reputation. Utilizing a balanced approach to decorating will result in a happy medium that expresses good taste, success, and comfort while avoiding pretensions.

THE WAITING ROOM

A seven-year-old girl comes home from school and tells her mother, "A boy in my class asked me to play doctor." "Oh, dear," the mother nervously sighed. "What happened, honey?" "Nothing. He made we wait forty-five minutes and then double-billed my insurance company."

Patients deplore waiting. The more apprehensive, aggravated, or inconvenienced they feel about seeing the doctor, the more volatile they become. While doctors with great bedside manner can often melt away patient hostility by entering the room with a resounding gracious welcome, it doesn't completely remove the bad taste garnered by the wait. Furthermore, the staff will resent the doctor, as they often feel the brunt of the patients' wrath.

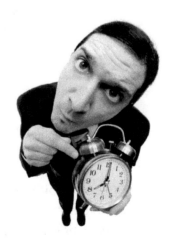

Some patients will actually leave an office, never to return, due to excessive wait times. The doctor with that great bedside manner may never have the chance to win over those patients. To avoid this type of occurrence, your goal should be to see every patient on time. Realistically, this is not always possible. Human interaction and medical treatment can be unpredictable. Some patients have more complicated problems and others need more time to understand the essentials of their case. Optimal care is the goal that supersedes punctuality, so it is a forgone conclusion that you will be running late much of the day.

As a specialist who sees a vast number of emergency patients in a field that often presents unpredictable treatment needs, I sympathize with doctors who run behind schedule. There are, however, methods to control the schedule so your office runs with the same precision seen in top service industries that have to process vast numbers of customers. Those who utilize these simple techniques will have the best reputation for all the little nuances that make patients think you have a great office.

Truth in Scheduling

If your office is always running behind, or if a patient asks how long a visit usually takes when they call to make an appointment, a truthful estimate goes a long way in preventing bad feelings. Patients appreciate knowing that two hours are needed for a visit allowing them to plan the rest of their day. It is always better to overestimate. A disclaimer should always be noted:

MR. SMITH
"I need to know how long this visit will take so I can adjust my schedule accordingly."

RECEPTIONIST
"I can't tell you exactly how long your visit with us will take because we, on occasion, have to deal with emergency patients. It would be best if you allot two hours from start to finish, though it usually doesn't take that long."

Many offices offer a time allotment based on the perfect day. Days don't always turn out to be perfect and the complaints of the disappointed patient only make it worse.

When a patient indicates they can't, or prefer not, to wait, it is best to offer them the first appointment in the morning or after lunch since those are the times with the least chance of being behind.

Catch-up Time Slots

To reduce the snowball effect of running behind schedule, you need to manage your time appropriately. This involves a realistic schedule you can handle with catch-up time incorporated. You should be able to figure out, with reasonable accuracy, how many emergencies you can expect on an ongoing basis. By leaving openings for these emergency patients you be less likely to run behind. Once you learn to manage your time efficiently, complex and unusual cases will no longer slow you down, and you will keep your day on schedule. Naturally, no matter how many slots you leave open, you need more, except on the days when you have too many – life is never predictable.

Knowing that time is the one commodity they cannot get more of, many doctors don't want to stand still for a moment. They tend to overbook and never allow for catch-up time. While they may see more patients, they keep everyone waiting inordinate amounts of time and rush through the day providing less than ideal treatment.

Off-Scheduling Appointments

When you cater to late patients, you run behind and make others wait even longer. Rather than fume every time someone is late, especially the same habitually tardy disorganized patients, you need to make rules that eliminate the effects of the inappropriate behavior. Consider *off-scheduling* habitually late patients from fifteen to thirty minutes before you expect to see them. This fifteen-minute difference between the time you tell the patient and the time you expect to see them helps keep you from waiting for late patients. It controls your anger.

Off-scheduling **new** patients works especially well, too. This affords time for them to find your office, fill out forms, and go to the bathroom for an excessive amount of time, a ritual that seems to be necessary, especially when you are waiting for the patient to be seated. The first appointment also allows you to see if the patient is on time and seems responsible. If they come late with no reasonable excuse and seem generally disinterested, you may want to continue off-scheduling them.

Off-scheduling helps to keep your schedule as fair as possible for the conscientious patients who respect your time by eliminating the wait caused by the inconsiderate patient. If you are never on time, you won't need any of these techniques since you are probably oblivious to time anyway.

Short Visit Priority

Most offices have **look visits**–certain types of appointments that can be classified as ultra-short. This visit is usually a follow-up exam to assess the progress of a treatment or response to medication. Making a patient wait an hour for a *look visit* is both inconsiderate and a manifestation of poor practice management. In general, give priority to all *look visits* – wait time should be ten minutes or less.

Make sure you have a way to determine which patients never let you out of the room. The **talker** may need special attention and can throw off your timing when you expect to have a *look visit* and it turns into *show and tell*. Cryptic notes on the patient chart can alert your secretary to make sure the appointment is scheduled properly for the *talker*, usually at the end of the day.

The assistant should screen each *look visit* patient before your entrance to make sure they are doing well. You don't want a surprise: "Doctor, I don't feel any better since you did the operation," because that kind of visit goes from the expected ultra-short *look visit* to the *okay, let's start all over visit.*

Obsessive Compulsive Providers

Don't feel compelled to complete every case on the spot. If you have a difficult case or a difficult patient, you may want to reschedule them to a later date when you have more time. Without offending your patient, you can suggest they have some tests completed or that you have to wait for test results.

As an example, you realize you're dealing with a chronic pain patient who needs a long evaluation and an extended amount of your time to explain the diagnosis and treatment protocol. Since you wanted blood tests to rule out organic pathology you can tell them you need to wait for the results. This allows you to schedule this patient for an extended second visit.

Once you learn to manage your time efficiently you avoid letting complex and unusual cases slow you down, and you will keep your day on schedule.

The Running Behind Apology

When patients have to wait for unexpected delays, make sure your staff apologizes for the wait, keeps the patients apprised of the approximate amount of time until they will be seen, and offers them the option to reschedule. Most patients will appreciate that you have their time at heart too.

Make sure your staff knows exactly what to say by giving them a rehearsed script: "Dr. Jones is in the middle of a very complex case and he is running behind. Once he is finished, he will devote all of his attention to your needs, but I just wanted you to know that he won't be able to see you for another half-hour. If this will affect your schedule adversely, we can reschedule your appointment."

When you enter the room, apologize and explain the nature of the delay. While it's not really your patient's business, they always think the worst: "He probably kept me waiting, while he spoke with his stockbroker."

The We Must Reschedule Apology

When you can't get out of the operating room, telling a patient who has waited an hour to see you that they will have to reschedule is not an easy task. You must make sure it's done properly. Obviously, you have to delegate tasks like this to your staff. They, too, should have a script that conveys your office policy and attitude. The way your staff handles this bad news is an extension of your bedside manner.

"The doctor won't be getting into the office today. We'll have to reschedule," is not the message you want to convey about the way you run your office. All too often, your staff is burnt out and gives that kind of message with little concern. There is a proper way to tell the patient.

"Mrs. Jones, (always use a name to show personal respect and concern) I'm terribly sorry, but Dr. Smith had an emergency come up at the hospital and he won't be able to get here for hours. I appreciate how you have waited so patiently, and again I am so sorry, but we are going to have to reschedule your appointment. Dr. Smith takes every patient's time seriously and he wanted me to personally apologize for this inconvenience."

When there is a waiting room full of patients, have the announcement made to all of them at once. To minimize the negative effect of situations like waiting with the possibility of rescheduling, it's a great idea to make sure patients know in advance that the nature of your practice necessitates such inconveniences. It should be stated clearly in your office brochure and on a *visible* sign posted in the waiting room.

Waiting room Sign For Offices That Occasionally Need to Reschedule Patients Unexpectedly

The nature of the practice of obstetrics often results in unexpected emergencies. While we try our best to be on time, the health and wellbeing of every patient comes first and foremost before being on schedule. We do hope you understand when you have to wait or are inconvenienced by rescheduling an appoint-

ment. When it is your turn, you will want the doctor's fullest time and attention, too.

Whenever a patient is rescheduled, it should be clearly noted in the chart so the doctor can be sure to apologize the next time the patient is seen:

DOCTOR

"Mary, I wanted to apologize and thank you for your understanding last week when I couldn't make it in to see you. I had a complex case at the hospital. Thank you again for your understanding."

In practices that require seeing emergencies on a regular basis make sure patients are aware of inconveniences that may arise by posting a *visible* sign.

Waiting Room Sign For Emergency Care Practices

The nature of our practice requires that we see emergencies. As a result, waiting to be seen by the doctor is sometimes necessary. We appreciate your understanding and know that when you need emergency care, we will be there to help you, while others will be inconvenienced.

The Floating Appointment

If you are notoriously running late, have a system set up where your secretary offers to call the patients as the time of their appointment nears in order to let them know how your schedule is flowing with an option to postpone the appointment.

The following are some excellent techniques to reduce the perception of a long wait:

Staged Waiting

Move patients from the waiting room to the treatment room in a manner that lets them wait in each space for around half of the wait time. While fifteen minutes in both places is still thirty minutes, it is perceived as less of a wait.

Occupying the Patient

Current magazines in the waiting room, as well as in each treatment room, are the most effective, cost-efficient way to keep your patients happy and distracted. Have a variety of magazines that will appeal to your entire patient base. Outdated magazines make you look cheap and careless. Have your staff dispose of the old or tattered issues regularly.

Television in the waiting room (and even in the treatment rooms) helps make the time go by. With the advent of digital video networks, companies may provide televisions for your waiting room that offer entertaining educational content. Utilize these free services as long as the content isn't too commercial in nature.

Cell Phones

Many doctors' offices and healthcare facilities don't let patients use cell phones while they wait. Since the cell phone may keep the patient busy and offer them some level of productivity, you should allow the use of cell phones, as long as it doesn't interfere with your activities and annoy other patients. You may want to suggest that the patient use the cell phone just outside the office. You can have your assistant get them when you are ready.

Partners and Associates

The Consummate ENT
I spoke with a number of patients who I referred to a
particular ENT and every one of them made the same
comment: "He is the nicest guy in the world. Thank you
so much for sending me to him." Those who had any
type of surgical procedure would go on about how he
called them at home several times during their recov-
ery to make sure they were well. It is that type of con-
nection that makes patients love you.
That's great bedside manner.

Unfortunately, it's not enough. Two patients told me
they never got to see him because the secretaries of-
fended them. When they called for appointments, the
doctor was booked out so far that they decided to
see someone more accommodating. So here we have
the most amazing doctor who doesn't realize he is
too busy and losing patients, or making them wait
so long to see him that their health could be jeopar-
dized. When I discussed the problem with him and
suggested an associate or partner, he had no interest.

In the final analysis, scheduling too many patients is the main cause of inordinate wait times. While you can't make as much money seeing fewer patients, your quality of life (and theirs) will improve. You must recognize when you work too hard, you damage your practice, your health and your personal relationships, and put your patients at risk.

It seems rather simple to remedy scheduling problems, just stop scheduling so many patients. Unfortunately, many health-care providers fall prey to financial pressures. They have all the excuses, including, "The HMO pays so little that I have to see a hundred patients a day to make ends meet." While there may be some truth to that, more often it's the new house, the sports car, and all the other goodies we work so hard for that need to be paid off.

In a consumer-oriented society, everyone wants the good things in life. You went to school for many years and studied while everyone else was having fun; finally it's your turn. Now you have a way to bill for services and you're willing to see a hundred patients a day. If you do, your reputation and bedside manner will suffer. Greed has no place in the practice of health-care sciences.

A partner or an associate will help alleviate the overwhelming patient load a doctor with the great bedside manner is sure to have.

Jeff was complaining to his friend Biff that love-making with his wife was becoming routine and boring. "Get creative, Jeff. Break up the monotony. Why don't you try playing doctor for an hour?
That's what I do," Biff said.
"Sounds great," Jeff replied, "but how do you make it last for an hour?"
"Hell, just keep her in the room waiting for fifty-five minutes!" replied Biff.

POLITICS AND RELIGION

Saint Peter had a terrible cold, so he asked Jesus if he
could have the day off to go to the doctor.
Jesus said, "Sure, I'll watch the Pearly Gates for you." It
was a slow day and at the end of the day an old man
with white hair approached the gates.
"May I enter the Kingdom of Heaven?"
Jesus replied, "We'd love to have you, but tell me what
you've done to earn your space here among the good?"
"I am but a simple carpenter, however my son was very
special. I raised him to be a carpenter too, but a mi-
raculous transformation came over him and to this day
all love him." Jesus smiled and jumped up, "Father!"
The old man opened his arms, "Pinocchio!"

Never discuss controversial issues. Diversity of thought is not conducive to endearing relationships with your patients. Your position as a doctor provides a soapbox you should avoid mounting. While it may be tempting to proselytize and persuade, you will offend more than you convert.

If a patient asks your opinion on any hot-button issue, tell them you never discuss politics or religion. Even if you know and agree with their political views, a patient in the next room (who's vehemently opposed to your beliefs) could overhear your conversation and find a new practitioner.

Since most people will not take the advice of the last two paragraphs, they should at least be armed with the proper rules of engagement when they venture into deep waters. While it is best to avoid discussing politics and religion, if you know where and when to discuss such taboo things you can develop some strong bonds with certain patients. The trick to *where* and *when* really comes down to *with whom* and *what* you should discuss. There is nothing more binding than to know that the other person embraces your politics or religion. There is also nothing more divisive that knowing you disagree with the other person's politics or religion. This means you have to know what the other person believes before you speak or you will get into trouble. If you don't know your patients, don't get started on controversial issues.

Here is an example of how it works. Whenever you treat law enforcement people, discuss how weak we are on crime, how the cops' hands are being tied, and how lawyers are screwing up everything. Of course when treating convicts, discuss the excesses of police brutality, how the death penalty is not a deterrent, and how mandatory sentences are just not fair to the criminal class. You get the idea.

Conversation with patients is rarely about politics and religion. More often your patients will enjoy conversation regarding everyday things you may have in common. If you treat many hunters, they will love your hunting stories and feel a particular closeness. Golf conversation is contagious between golfers. If your patient is wearing a Greenpeace button, sure, go ahead and tell them about how you bombed a fishing boat to protect the dolphins; it can't hurt.

Most small communities are rather homogenous. Quite often, everyone in a small town belongs to the same house of worship and they maintain memberships in the same clubs. This affords you the opportunity to have common beliefs, goals, and aspirations. If you know your people, you can discuss anything as long as you agree with them.

FORBIDDEN VOCABULARY

The Top Ten Things You Should Never Say During Surgery

10. "Don't worry. I think it is sharp enough."
9. "Nurse, did this patient sign the organs donation card?"
8. "Damn! Page eighty-four of the manual is missing!"
7. "Everybody stand back! I lost a contact lens!"
6. "Hand me that...uh...that uh.....thingie."
5. "Better save that. We'll need it for the autopsy."
4. "What do you mean 'She doesn't need this part?'"
3. "Whoa, wait a minute, if this is his spleen, then what's that?"
2. "Accept this sacrifice, O Great Lord of Darkness."
1. "Oops!"

There are countless ways you can make the patient experience better by using language that neither scares nor confuses. Many words should be stricken from office jargon or substituted with euphemisms. The more innocuous the terms used, the better the patient will feel about the procedure. Each practitioner needs a personal list of taboo words and field-specific terminology.

There are good and bad ways to give patients information. In general, avoid technical terms. While these terms make the doctor appear learned, they are often confusing to the patient suddenly required to learn a new vocabulary in order to understand a complicated procedure. Technical terms often sound sterile and may frighten patients who have visions of dreaded procedures being performed on them or loved ones. Patients appreciate plain English.

I was enjoying lunch at the local deli when the owner, who liked to hang out with the doctors, told us a story. He had a surgical procedure under local anesthesia. It was a common procedure I do in my office. He told us how, during the operation, the surgeon told him he was "grinding the bone" and he nearly passed out. I was a young doctor at the time and I remember his words to this day. At that moment, I realized there are good and bad ways to give patients information. If you get it right, your clear and simple explanations are just another manifestation of great bedside manner.

Whenever I do that particular surgery and get to the part where I need to use the drill to remove some bone, I tell the patient, "I'm smoothing off your tooth. Don't let the sound of the drill bother you."

Smooth is better than *grind*, and *tooth* is better than *bone*. That's the right way to say it, even if it's not entirely true. By utilizing proper words and explanations, the patient has a pleasant experience. If the procedures you do are performed using general anesthesia, the rules of forbidden vocabulary don't apply unless you believe that the unconscious patient still hears what's going on.

Some patients like to know what's going on, and all patients like to know when you will be finished with the procedure. You have to decide which type of patient you have. If the patient says, "Doc, do what you have to do, just don't tell me about it." They really mean it, and you should limit your talk to things unrelated to the procedure except for keeping them abreast of how much longer you have to go.

Since everyone wants to get out as soon as possible, try to be fairly honest in your time to completion appraisal. Use words of encouragement often and link your patient's good behavior with being able to get finished faster. This type of praise gets the patient to work harder to help you get done quicker: "You are doing great and by being such a great patient you're helping me to get done faster." When you are on the last stage mention that too: "You are doing fine and we're on the last stage." Compliments make the patient feel good about themselves, they distract them from thinking about the procedure, and they keep them focused on the positive rather than imagining everything is going wrong.

In contrast to the patient who doesn't want to know anything, some patients like you to describe every detail of the procedure. For the inquisitive patient, you may tell them what you are doing but try not to be too graphic. You can still use innocuous terms like smoothing instead of drilling and tooth instead of bone.

Other patients want any type of conversation to get their mind off the procedure. To accomplish this goal, you may speak of simple matters like discussing an upcoming holiday, the weather, a recent or planned vacation, as well as throwing in a multitude of compliments for how well they are doing.

If you can't chew gum and walk, don't start talking to your patient while doing a procedure requiring your fullest attention. You should, however, explain to the patient why you may not be talking throughout the procedure, and that you'll try to keep them abreast of what's happening. "Some of this procedure requires that I concentrate, so I may not be able to talk too much while I'm working."

If you are going to tell the patient what you are doing, discretion is still warranted. You don't need an inquisitive patient fainting on you. Use simple lay terms like, "I'm removing the infection." That sounds much better than, "I'm scooping out the dead bone from your arm."

It is easy to forget what terms are technical when you use them on a daily basis. The word *tissue* may seem reasonable to use with patients, but for many they picture Kleenex when you use that word. Try skin or gum and they'll know what you mean.

"I'm making an *opening* to remove the infection," sounds much better than, "I'm *cutting you open* to remove the infection," or, "I'm making an *incision*," which sounds sterile, technical, and invasive.

Remove sounds better than *extracting*, or *pulling*. And for heaven's sake, they will have no idea what you're doing if you tell them you're *enucleating* the cyst *or debriding the lesion.*

Don't tell a patient they have to *go under the knife*. That term is grotesque and archaic. It should be banned from medical jargon. A knife has connotations of cutting and stabbing. It is much kinder to say, "You need an operation (or surgery)," or "We have to remove that little lump."

Never mention that you are working on muscles or bone. "I'm finishing up now," is much better than, "I'm reconnecting the muscles."

Words and phrases that confuse or scare the patient and some substitutes follow:

Irrigate/debride the wound = rinse the cut, or rinse out the opening.

Necrotic = bad stuff – "I'm going to remove the necrotic tissue," versus, "I'm going to remove the bad stuff." Yes, you went to medical school for all those years to talk like an idiot. A simple term like "bad stuff" makes some patients comfortable in the "down to earth" way you communicate with them. If you are uncomfortable with "bad stuff," you can use the term *infection* as it sounds professional without scaring. To *remove infection* sounds good to the patient.

Sutures are *stitches. Tissues* are either *gum* or *skin.*

Don't tell your assistant you need her to stop the *bleeding*; rather you need her to control the *flow.* The patient has no idea what is flowing and bleeding makes them think there is a problem. Telling your assistant to *irrigate or suction* is another cryptic way of telling them to suction excessive bleeding.

Orthopedic and oral surgeons use an instrument called a *bone cutter.* "Mary, pass the bone cutter," is not what most patients want to hear. Doctors with great bedside manner don't own bone cutters. They use trimmers; not bone trimmers, just plain old trimmers.

Some doctors use *chisels* during bone surgery. Most people would rather go to the doctor who uses *smoothers or files* rather than *chisels.* We don't use *mallets* or *hammers,* we use *tappers.* While you may use *clamps* I use *clips. Pliers* and *forceps* are *grippers,* and a *saw* can be a *linear file.* Make up whatever terms you must to convey a friendly environment.

Your patients shouldn't have an *atypical* infection (*lesion, anatomy,* etc.). They'd better understand and much rather have an *unusual* infection, or an *unusual shaped tooth.*

"*Exacerbations*" are "*flare-ups.*" "*Protracted*" is "*longstanding.*" "*Occult*" is "*hard to find or hidden.*" Never discuss the "*prognosis*" with your patients. Instead, you discuss *"the chance of this working out."* You never *"lay a flap,"* you *"lift the gum back."* Your patients appreciate plain English.

Pain is *discomfort, soreness,* or *an ache,* but don't avoid mentioning pain if there is a good chance the patient will experience some. You patients will worry more if you tell them there could be some discomfort and they have pain. It is actually better to have them expect the worst and be pleasantly surprised. You will never have a patient call you after hours worried that they had no pain after you told them they could have some.

Today, most patients know the term *scalpel.* Your patients should never hear that word from you. Say, "Pass the Bard-Parker fifteen," or your assistant can say, "Would you like the B-P fifteen?" This is merely a code for the brand and type scalpel. The patient should have no idea when or where you use a knife.

These are just a few ideas you can incorporate into your practice to make the patient experience better. Buy a small digital recorder and keep it available to record your next ten conversations with patients to see how well you communicate and the quality of your bedside manner. Keep your ears open and have your staff alert you to any terms they think need to be changed to make your practice the one everyone wants to go to for care.

FIRST NAMES, ENDEARING NAMES,
AND TOUCH

Each professional must decide how to address patients and how they would prefer to be titled. Some doctors strive for a casual office while others prefer formality. There is a way to have both and to please most everyone.

The way to greet patients varies from one geographic or socio-economic setting to another. As a rule of thumb, staff should address young patients (under thirty years of age) by first name and older patients (over thirty years of age) by surnames. Doctors may use first names for most patients under sixty years of age.

A twenty-year-old calling an eighty-year-old woman Sally may be offensive, just as a ten-year-old boy may not like being called Mr. Jones. You must be aware of generational differences and understand how respect is defined and interpreted.

While some doctors prefer introducing themselves by their first name, considering it a plus for bedside manner, it is inappropriate and should be avoided. A title defines the relationship, and calling doctors by first names degrades the doctor-patient relationship. Most patients want you to be the doctor. They look to the doctor for care and healing. Most patients aren't looking for a friend.

If staff members use your name repeatedly before you meet the patient, it precludes your need to be formal and you can offer a friendly, "Good morning," otherwise it is best to greet with your name attached, "Good morning, I'm Dr. Fleisher."

Some patients like to call their doctors by first name, probably because it makes them feel important. If a patient asks to call you by your first name, go along with the request to avoid appearing stuffy.

Using endearing names at the appropriate time is an easy way to express affability and compassion to your patients. This involves no learning or personality changes on your part other than picking the names and using them.

Be very careful in choosing endearing names. Sweetheart, baby, or honey could be considered sexist by many adults, while others appreciate the affection and concern it shows. These same names work well with children. To tell a frightened little girl, "You are doing great, sweetheart," is comforting and helpful in getting her through the procedure.

There are endearing names for different ages, personalities, socioeconomic groups and cultures. Decide upon the ones you are comfortable using. They should fit with your personality and demeanor. You don't want to overdo it either. Most people do not appreciate over solicitousness. Using endearing names at the right time is an easy way to improve your bedside manner.

If you are the quiet retiring type, saying *hey baby* may not be the best choice. Likewise, *hey baby* may not be right for a seventy-year-old during a routine gynecological exam. Yet *hey baby* may work just fine for the cosmetic surgeon practicing in Beverly Hills. Buckaroo works very well for a little fellow around five years of age, while an accountant may think you are nuts if you call him by that endearing name. The following list offers endearing names most suited for professional practice along with suggested uses.

ENDEARING NAME	GENDER	AGE	SITUATION
Partner, Buckaroo, Pal, Cowboy, Soldier,	Male	<12	Greeting, Compliments, Recognizing Distress
Buddy, Pal	Male	< 55	Greeting, Compliments, Recognizing Distress
Friend, my friend	Male Female	>15 <55	Greeting, Compliments, Recognizing Distress
Sir	Male		Formal Greeting, Formal Discussion, Recognizing Distress
Partner, Champ	Male	<25	Greeting, Compliments, Recognizing Distress
Cupcake, Honeybunch, Baby Doll, Doll Baby, Honey Bun, Cutie, Gorgeous, Beautiful	Female	<12	Greeting, Compliments, Recognizing Distress
Darling, Sweetheart	Female	<55 <12*	Compliments, Recognizing Distress – to be used with **caution**, as some consider these terms inappropriate and sexist except for use with children*
Ma'am, Madam, Dear	Female	>30	Formal Greeting, Formal Discussion, Recognizing Distress
Dear	Female	Any Age	Can Be Both Endearing or Demeaning for Greeting, Compliments, Recognizing Distress

During treatment you should try to use an endearing name whenever you receive nonverbal communication, i.e. wincing in pain, cringing, sudden tenseness.

Mary shows some signs of distress during treatment. You say, "You are doing so well, darling, and we are just about done." You read and acknowledged that Mary is having some distress, you offer comfort by telling her it is almost over, and you provide the endearment by using the term *darling*. This response to Mary is the difference between a doctor with great bedside manner and the doctor who is busy performing a procedure and completely oblivious to the patient.

Certain names work better with different socioeconomic groups. *Pal* is more of a blue-collar name while *friend* may be better for the doctor who is your patient.

The use of endearing names should be avoided upon initially meeting an adult patient while it is very acceptable and helpful in developing a fast bond with a child. When you walk in the room of a child, greeting them with a, "Hi there soldier (cowboy, buckaroo, or buddy)," works fine. Upon greeting an adult male patient, saying, "Good morning, Mr. Jones (sir or John)," is a better way to start the relationship.

Once you begin treatment, you can switch to *pal, buddy, friend*, or *my friend* if your relationship and personality, and the personality of the patient, warrant such familiarity. "You are doing great, my friend!"

"We're just about done, buddy" works much better than ignoring the patient's body language or than using the patient's formal name: "We're just about done, Mr. Jones." The tone of the endearing name does just what it is supposed to do; endear you to the patient.

Except for some stuffy patients, you can never go wrong using a first name, especially in a matter of duress. For those who find it difficult to use endearing names, try to use first names, often, to convey friendliness and ease tension.

"Do you need a little more Novocain, Mary?" works much better than, "Do you need more Novocain, madam?" Sir and madam are too formal. First names are friendlier than last names, and while there is nothing wrong with using the first or last name, in most cases the endearing name makes for a higher level of connection.

Besides being too formal, using the terms *madam, ma'am* and *sir* may be interpreted as expressing disdain. Addressing the patient as dear, madam, ma'am, or sir is often used when the health-care provider is frustrated, or otherwise fed up with the patient and will engender hostile feelings. These terms can also be used in a respectful manner, so don't totally avoid them if they work for you, just recognize the tone you use.

"Are you alright, dear?" is fine while, "Dear, this can't be hurting that bad," sounds condescending and hostile.

Physical contact with patients can convey the highest level of caring, comfort, and compassion. The most common form of physical contact is the handshake. This gesture helps to form an immediate bond. While you socialize with professionals all the time as part of your training and station in life, it may be difficult for you to understand that patients often think of doctors as special people and to take the time to shake hands is often appreciated more than many realize.

The hand on the shoulder and pat on the back are other ways to convey friendship and good wishes. The hand on the shoulder works well when a patient becomes upset over something they realize is out of anyone's control. A hug works for cases where you have to deliver bad news and the patient is about to cry. You have to be careful with hugs, as sometimes the patient may not expect, or want, this type of contact. If you have years of history with the patient, physical gestures are often more welcome.

All physical contact should be avoided when you are alone with the patient. While it never used to be a concern, the last thing you want is an accusation that you were trying to make sexual advances toward your patient.

BODY LANGUAGE

Most people want health-care providers who communicate well and offer some level of conversation. Despite this obvious fact, some doctors don't converse with their patients, and more importantly they don't communicate at a most critical moment: when the patient is in distress or in pain. While every doctor responds to the screaming patient, only the perceptive observer reads body language to help him or her respond to less clearly expressed patients' needs.

Body language is a form of nonverbal communication ranging from the easy-to-read (laughing and crying: both of which could represent happiness, fear, apprehension or pain) to the more subtle manifestations that require astute observation and impeccable interpretation. It is the understated messages that require a higher level of awareness.

For health-care providers the most important messages conveyed by body language regard pain, fear, anxiety, confusion, mistrust, financial concerns, and the acceptance or refusal of treatment options. Failure to read these signs can adversely affect your relationship with your patients.

The doctor who can tell when patients don't understand them, don't trust their opinion, or have no intention of following their treatment plan have a tremendous advantage. They can adjust their conversation in order to address and remedy patient concerns. Doctors who know what their patients think and how they feel practice at a higher level of competence.

Body Language Considerations

Body language doesn't always tell you what you think it does. Laughter may be a friendly gesture, an expression of joy or a manifestation of fear and anxiety. The doctor must find out what patients are experiencing in order to help them effectively. You can use simple greetings to open the door for dialogue that gets your patient to offer more information.

Fear and Pain

When you walk into a room and the patient is wiping tears from their eyes, establish immediately if they are in pain, and if so, how much of the tearing is pain and how much is fear. Ignoring the tears all together is interpreted as a lack of compassion and not the way to practice medicine.

Consider a humorous greeting to establish an immediate bond and it will help to alleviate patient apprehension:

DOCTOR
"Are those tears of joy because you're so happy to see me?"

This allows the patient to explain the tears without feeling pressured and opens the door for gentle questioning. If the patient is in pain, they will usually proceed to tell you how much pain they have.

If they are tears of fear and apprehension, they will usually chuckle through the tears, ignore you, or begin to tell you how frightened they are to see you.

With one humorous question you respond to the patient's obvious body language in a compassionate manner.

A variation for the tear-wiping patient:

DOCTOR
"Correct me if I'm wrong, but tears like that tell me
you'd rather be somewhere else right now."

You walk in the room and the patient has their head in their hands. This tells you the patient is in pain, fearful, annoyed, miserable, or praying. It is your job to find out what they are experiencing:

DOCTOR
"If you're in the middle of praying that you were some-where else right now, I can come back later."

Variation:

DOCTOR
"It looks like I caught you in the middle of some deep meditation. I can come back later if you wish."

The Miserable Patient

DOCTOR
"Good morning."

The patient doesn't respond. Others may offer an unfriendly response to your greeting. That's their subtle way of telling you they are angry. You continue:

DOCTOR
"You don't seem very happy to see me. Is it the color of my scrubs?"

By asking a direct, funny question, the patient will be forced to respond, and they will often chuckle and explain why they are miserable. The answer usually involves pain or fear, but be ready when they say:

PATIENT
"Well, you kept me waiting two hours."

Make sure you have a catchy response for such complaints to regain the patient's goodwill:

DOCTOR
"So it isn't the color of my scrubs. I am terribly sorry I kept you waiting. Unfortunately, we had many emergencies and every patient gets my fullest attention before I can move on."

Most patients will accept an apology, but realize that there are some patients who will continue to grunt, act moody, or stay uncomfortably quiet. You can't please everyone.
Other humorous options include:

DOCTOR
"I would have been in here sooner if my parole officer just stopped asking all those questions."

Pause:
Actually, I am terribly sorry I kept you waiting. Unfortunately, we had many emergencies and every patient gets my fullest attention before I can move on.

Or:

DOCTOR
"I would have been in sooner, but you know how hangovers can last longer than you expect."

Pause:
"Actually, I am terribly sorry I kept you waiting. Unfortunately, we had many emergencies and every patient gets my fullest attention before I can move on."

These lines will soften the angry patients or they will get up and walk out. If they walk out, you're lucky. You didn't want to see that person anyway.

Of course, you can respond with just an apology if you don't wish to try the bold comedic style:

DOCTOR
"I'm terribly sorry to keep you waiting. Unfortunately, I had a patient who was up all night in pain and they needed some extra attention. I'm sure you'd want me to provide you with the same level of service."

Even when the patient doesn't tell you they are mad because you made them wait, you have to read the body language. You know you are an hour late and if the patient acts cold, that's enough for you to use the apology without them saying they are upset.

Treatment Pain

During the course of a routine procedure or injection, patients often make a face, squirm, wince, or otherwise tell you they are uncomfortable. It is imperative that you acknowledge their statement. While you may have prepared them for the procedure, you still need to respond to their nonverbal statement. A thoughtful, "I know this hurts," or "I'm sorry this is so uncomfortable," or *"We're almost done,"* is the acknowledgement the patient wants to hear.

They now know you are the best doctor because you responded to their statement, unlike those other doctors who ignore them.

Financial Concerns

You mention the fee for a procedure that isn't covered by the patient's insurance and they roll their eyes, or you may see a less perceptible facial movement such as the eyes opening wide, or the eyebrows rising. Now is the time to respond to their nonverbal communication.

DOCTOR
"Mary, I know that's a lot of money, but the benefit…"

By responding to the unspoken word, you acknowledge that you understand Mary's concern, and that you are compassionate to her financial considerations.

Treatment Acceptance

When you are attuned to reading body language, you will be able to tell when the patient is not interested in accepting your treatment plan, and this affords you the opportunity to add some commentary that might change their mind.

After a lengthy explanation of your proposed treatment, the fact that a patient doesn't say much isn't necessarily a rejection of your plan. Patients are often quiet as a result of fear, confusion, or they may just have limited personality. You have to ask them if they have any questions. Don't be afraid to ask:

DOCTOR
"So, what would you like to do?"

If they are noncommittal and tell you they need to "think it over," you should show your concern by concluding the visit:

DOCTOR
"That would be best. I want you to make your decision
when you have had a chance to think it over so you won't
feel that you are rushing into this. If you have any questions, I want you to give us a call and we'll try to clarify anything to help you make the right choice."

That sounds a lot nicer and more compassionate than, "I think you're making a mistake by not choosing to do this right now." The only time to give a stern warning about starting a procedure is when the patient's health is in immediate jeopardy by delaying treatment.

Patients who are undecided very often despise the pushy doctor and will never return. They interpret the pushy doctor as greedy and more concerned with self-interests. High-pressure tactics will not convince the fiscally responsible patient who can't afford treatment, and they will not return when they can.

You have to be sophisticated in your interpretation as reading body language is an art and takes years to learn to do well. It offers you a tremendous advantage in knowing what your patients want to tell you, but don't in the conventional manner.

While patients don't actually recognize all the reasons they like certain doctors, the doctor who addresses fears, anxiety, treatment choices, and financial concerns they don't have to verbalize is the doctor they want to see all the time.

Don't forget that body language is a two way street. You may be sending the wrong signals when you make a facial expression, smirk, sneer or even look at your watch. You may inadvertently tell the patient you are disinterested, annoyed, impatient or running behind. Don't make repeated eye contact with your assistant or nurse. This could make the patient think your assistant is making negative gestures about them. These are just a few of the messages better-kept private. Patients may sense that you have no interest in their care or that you are burned out.

Try to communicate to your patients that you love what you do. Try to act enthusiastic about every case. Compliment your work and make sure your staff knows that when they compliment an outcome the patient appreciates it. Never let a patient see you sweat or struggle. Make every effort to make everything you do look easy, even if you have to take acting lessons.

DELIVERING BAD NEWS

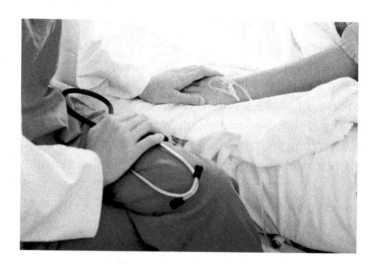

A man goes to his doctor for a complete checkup. He hasn't been feeling well and wants to find out if he's ill. After the checkup the doctor comes out with the results of the examination.
"I'm afraid I have some bad news. You're dying and you don't have much time," the doctor says.
"Oh no, that's terrible. How long have I got?"
the man asks.
"Ten..." says the doctor.
"Ten? Ten what? Months? Weeks? What?!" he asks desperately.
"9...8...7..."

An ICU nurse says that when there is bad news to deliver, doctors often lack the bedside manner to deliver it well. "Doctors are sometimes not so great at it and they leave us standing there to deal with the family. I give them a hug because I'm that type of person. We don't have any formal program to tell the family. Of course, after the fact, they can see grief counselors. There was this one guy who didn't make it after open-heart surgery. We were just waiting for him to die and even after we unplugged everything he still held on. We couldn't figure out what was holding him on. All the while the family was at his bedside – all but a twin son who didn't get there until much later. Once he arrived, he held his father's hand and at that moment he passed. There was something special about that and while we can't explain it, there is more to life than we understand. The family was grateful that we stayed with them as long as necessary."

It's never easy delivering bad new whether it's as mundane as explaining why a minor procedure didn't work as expected, or as sad as telling the family the patient died.

In a litigious society, the way bad news is announced can be the difference between the successful delivery of a message versus the messenger being shot. As unfortunate and callous as it may sound, avoiding litigation is a reality in a world that assumes if something went wrong it was the doctor's fault.

A Gastroenterologist's Experiences
"I once had six deaths in 24 hours in ICU. There is no right way to tell the family. I use the euphemism: 'I'm sorry, but your mother moved on.' Quite often I would hear the loved ones say things like:

'Did you see my mom's soul go to heaven?' I would
reply: 'God hasn't given me the privilege to see or
understand that kind of thing.' The physician is in
a no-win situation. How can you console a mother
who lost a daughter? Never say, 'I know how you
feel.' It's better to say, 'I know you feel bad.'"

"I had to tell an eighty-year-old woman and her
daughter that her husband (the daughter's father)
had died. Not a moment after I told the wife, she
passed out right there on the floor and died. I initi-
ated a code and we tried to revive her, but to no
avail. I looked up to the daughter and said, 'Please
don't die on me.' It sounded so cruel, but she under-
stood and kindly said, 'Don't worry, I'm all right.'"

Many times people say they are going to sue the doctor when they have a loss. They often don't understand or believe the doctor's explanation, and once they institute a suit, the explanation will come in a long, tiring, brutal, and hostile environment of depositions and testimony. If complications are explained in a compassionate, understandable manner, the courtroom can be avoided, and the aggrieved will better cope with their loss.

The most difficult bad news involves telling the family the patient died. "I'm terribly sorry, Mary, but I just killed you mother," is not the way you would ever deliver bad news, but you can be sure that's the message the personal injury attorney is going to deliver to the jury of laymen who will decide your fate. While compassion has to be the utmost concern at the time of delivering news of loss, you also must be concerned with protecting yourself.

Since blame is the essence of personal injury law, you must make sure you assign blame to the patient, unless you truly performed an act of malpractice and wish to make such a pronouncement.

Assuming you did nothing wrong, it is best to begin by establishing a rapport with any of the family members you may not already know. This is especially true for the emergency room physician, who often meets the family for the first time to deliver the news that a loved one died.

You need to introduce yourself and determine to whom you are speaking:

DOCTOR
"I'm Doctor Smith."

In most instances the person will tell you
who they are, if not, you ask:

DOCTOR
"How are you related to Joan?"

You put out your hand, take their hand in both of yours. This immediately shows concern and compassion. You repeat this for each person you need to know.

DOCTOR
"Please, let's sit down and let me explain."

Once everyone is seated:

DOCTOR
"We did everything we could, but Joan's injuries were
just too extensive and she didn't make it."

Often the loved one will try to get the bad news by shouting, "Did she die?" It is best to respond to the demand since this personality doesn't want to wait for protocol.

Notice the blame is placed upon the injuries, and you avoided the harsh sound of *dead* or *died* by using the euphemism "didn't make it." You now must allow time for the response, which will often be hysteria. If the person grabs you, you hug them and tell them how terribly sorry you are and that you wish there was something more you could say or do to make things better.

The more difficult situation arises when you have to tell the family their loved one died in a case where it was never expected. Probably the worst such scenario is when the patient dies during routine cosmetic surgery. Again, blame should be placed upon the patient.

Every doctor knows there is risk associated with surgery and general anesthesia. These risks are supposed to be spelled out in the informed consent and that consent is your best protection. Though the patient consents to the procedure and is supposed to understand the risk, that doesn't mean they, or their family, will not still attempt to sue the doctor.

Patients usually don't sue doctors they love and trust. While the patient may have loved you and would never sue, that doesn't mean their family feels the same way. It is at this time that you have to establish the rapport, trust, and bond with the loved ones to prevent a lawsuit. Beyond protecting yourself, you should understand that the most important motive to establishing this relationship with the family is to help them deal with a most unfortunate event in their lives.

Defensive posturing is not compassionate and makes the doctor look suspect. It is best to explain the nature of surgical risk in the most lay fashion possible:

DOCTOR
"I have terrible news for you. Your wife had a bad reaction to the anesthesia and we couldn't revive her."

Most loved ones will respond to the euphemism:

FAMILY MEMBER
"You mean she died?"

DOCTOR
"I'm sorry."

It is imperative to stay with the family as long as is necessary. Rushing away without cause appears callous. If you are the emergency room physician and it's a busy day, you may have to excuse yourself, but you should make sure there is some protocol in your hospital to have a grief counselor, or nurse trained in dealing with these matters, take over once you have explained the situation. At that point you must explain that there is another emergency for which you are needed and introduce the counselor before you make your exit.

Never rush the family of the bereaved. Try to answer all the questions they may have. Always ask if there are any questions before you leave and say, "If there is anything else I can do for you please don't hesitate to give me a call." That offer to "give me a call" goes a long way toward making the patient, or the family, feel comfortable.

Now that you can tell a family member their loved one just died, everything else is easy. Maybe not. No one likes bad news, and when you have to deliver it, it's never pleasant for either party. Again, you must be prepared for any and all situations and have a script ready. No matter how trivial you think a loss may be, to a particular patient it could be devastating.

Failing Procedures

An Endodontist
"Telling patients a procedure failed is very uncomfortable for me. I always plan for failure when making a treatment plan. I tell the patient what we will have to do in the event that things don't go as planned. I explain the alternatives, risks, and costs. I want my patients to be comfortable with any outcome."

When a procedure fails, patients are at minimum disappointed, and others may exhibit hostility. Much of the reaction depends upon expectations, importance of the procedure, and financial loss. The loss of sight would be more disconcerting than the loss of a tooth. A loss involving a simple procedure with a high expectation for success is more upsetting than the failure of a procedure that had limited chance of success. And the failure of any procedure that required large out-of-pocket expense is less acceptable than the failing procedure fully covered by insurance.

All of these considerations must be addressed before treatment to avoid the bad feeling engendered when procedures fail. By preparing before the failure, delivering the bad news is much easier and preserves your relationship with the patient.

Besides the written informed consent, the doctor should deliver the oral consent and address all the possibilities of complications and chance of failure. If presented in a friendly, non-threatening manner, treatment acceptance will be high and disappointment minimized when treatment fails.

Most reasonable patients will understand a failing procedure and accept the need to move on. Some might question you about a refund. There are two schools of thought on this issue. You can offer some type of refund, best tied into an alternative treatment or you can revert to your informed consent where you prepared the patient so well they shouldn't even consider asking for a refund. In spite of the best preparation, telling the patient who never understood your presentation that there is no refund, and they will now have to pay for the new device, is not well received. Which doctor are you going to love? I think we all know the answer.

To make a fair settlement, you can offer to apply the funds from the failed procedure towards an alternative or you can tell them they will get some sort of discount. Patients will be much happier if they feel they didn't lose everything. While you will take a loss for a minimal amount, you will have a very happy patient. Since failures should be an uncommon occurrence, you can afford to be nice.

Some practitioners feel that offering a discount or refund is tantamount to admitting guilt. While that is a concern, most patients do not think that way. Even if they tried to use the refund against you in a lawsuit, good records and documentation that you are making a hardship adjustment will look favorable for you in the courtroom, though you'll not likely get there.

Many doctors spend thousands of dollars marketing their practices and they are reluctant to make an adjustment when things go wrong. The goodwill generated by a patient who doesn't have to pay twice for the same thing is worth many times more than marketing costs. The badmouthing that takes place when the disgruntled patient pays twice costs even more.

Besides death and failing procedures, there are lesser bits of bad news that need attention as well if you want to run the premier professional practice. It is bad enough that health-care providers are often behind schedule and keep patients waiting; sometimes hospital emergencies require them to miss appointments. The chapter on the waiting room addresses such problems.

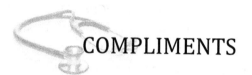

COMPLIMENTS

Doctor: "You have acute appendicitis."
Blonde: "I came here for medi-
cal help, not compliments."

Everyone likes to be complimented. People feel good about themselves when they receive a compliment and they feel good about the person giving the compliment.

An ER Doctor: "No one likes to be told they are a ter-
rible patient. It is very tempting to agree with the
patient who announces that they are the 'worst pa-
tient you'll ever see.' While they may be right, they
prefer to hear you say, 'Oh, you're not anywhere
near the worst patient I've ever seen. As a matter of
fact you are doing rather well considering the cir-
cumstances.' After agreeing with some of the worst
patients imaginable, I found that I hurt their feel-
ings. An ounce of honey is much better at getting any
semblance of cooperation than a cup of vinegar."

Giving compliments is not always a natural behavior. Some people never have a nice word to say and others offer compliments so readily that they have limited credibility. The use of compliments to enhance bedside manner requires observational skills to find the perfect words and the knowledge of when to use them. You don't want to be thought of as disingenuous. If you become attuned to peoples' body language and behavior, and understand when and how a compliment works, you will find the right words to say.

Appearance Compliments

The observant practitioner will notice the patient who takes great pride in their dress and knows that they truly appreciate recognition for all the time and effort and money that went into their outfit and accessories.

The elderly man or woman may wear a nice hat or scarf that coordinates perfectly with their outfit. Recognition of the effort expended in preparing for a visit with the doctor by offering a compliment is greatly appreciated.

DOCTOR
"My, what a lovely outfit, Mrs. Jones."

Those few words just made someone's day, and they will love you forever. The astute practitioner recognizes all sorts of things like this, and while the object of the compliment doesn't have to please your personal taste, the offering is still very effective.

While you may not personally relish tattoos, whenever someone has a particularly large one, consider a compliment. They saved three weeks salary to get this demon from hell breathing lightning bolts from oversized nostrils painted indelibly on their calf, and they wear shorts in the dead of winter to it show off. You better believe they love that you noticed the masterpiece (who could miss it) and told them how you really like the vivid colors.

You should make a concerted effort to give physical compliments whenever they are apropos. Offer compliments about hairstyle (your hair looks great!) or color (you have the most lovely blonde hair);

clothing and accessories (that dress is stunning on you; I love those jeans; that is such a great pocketbook); eye color (you have the most beautiful blue eyes); and anything you think the patient takes pride in. Just be careful not to make your friendly compliments too personal, so they can't be mistaken for sexual advances.

Behavior Compliments

Even more appreciated are compliments about how the patient performs at the visit. This form of encouragement goes a long way in helping your patients through difficult procedures. The more frightened the patient, the more they appreciate being told how well they are doing. Not only will they love the compliment, they will actually try to live up to your praise–making your job easier.

Every patient who works with you deserves compliments throughout the treatment. What doctors eventually take for granted because they do it everyday may be a monumental difficulty for the average patient.

Here are just a few compliments you could offer throughout the day.

You are doing great. You are the best patient I've seen today. I can't believe how well you are doing. I can't believe you never had root canal therapy before. I've seen an awful lot of patients over the years and not many are as good as you. Mary, do you believe how well Jim is doing? (Mary is your assistant).

There are several funny compliments presented in the chapter on comedy that work fine, too. If you stay attuned to people's appearance and behavior, you can learn to compliment many of the things that make your patients feel good.

PROFESSIONAL BURNOUT

Top Five Signs You're Suffering Burnout
5. You're so tired you forget to go to sleep.
4. Your five year old kid says, "Good morning," and you yell, "What's good about it?"
3. Your secretary says you're being robbed and you run out to confront the robber, expecting it to be less stressful that dealing with Mrs. Nudnik.
2. You wake up and your bed is on fire, but you're so tired you go back to sleep.
1. You think how relaxing it would be if you were in jail right now.

Everyone is entitled to have a bad day... except people in service industries. How many times have you experienced a service provider having a bad day, causing you to say, "I'll never go back to that place again"? We all have bad days; the problem is that no one wants to know about your bad day. When you meet a miserable service provider for the first and only time, you may have no idea how won-

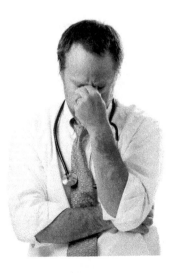

derful they are on all other days and you really don't care. Most people are only concerned about today.

For the healthcare provider with the great bedside manner it is important to avoid showing the effects of the bad day, and even more imperative is the need to stay focused and avoid becoming burned out.

In essence, burnout is physical or emotional exhaustion, especially as a result of long-term stress. It doesn't take a lot of years to become a victim of burnout when trying to seek perfection in an imperfect world, dealing with difficult patients, lackluster staff, demanding colleagues, and insurance carriers denying payments, all the while worrying about being sued and losing your home. Just about this time you should consider a career change. Yes, you should go ahead and open that candy store.

Much burnout comes from a "too busy" practice. Trying to see too many patients is physically demanding, and deep down inside there is the mental anguish of knowing you aren't performing the type of care you are capable of providing. Rationalization often surfaces and you tell yourself: *the way the HMO pays me, the patients are lucky I have time to say hello.* You worry about maintaining your income and you cut corners even further. Don't let your practice run your life and corrupt your values.

A busy neurosurgeon gives this advice to new doctors to prevent burnout:

"Make sure they are associated with a group so they can have a life. Make sure they know the emergency room docs; who's good and experienced and who's not. Then you will be better able to know when something is a true emergency."

Diagnostic challenges, personal physical decline, dealing with difficult people and staff, as well as forces external to your practice (like family issues or even the classic midlife crisis) are strong catalysts for burnout.

At the opposite end of the spectrum is the practice that can barely pay the bills because the practitioner is lacking in business skills or people skills (poor bedside manner), or the location of the office is not ready for a fulltime practitioner. Not being busy enough can be just as bad as being too busy.

It's easy to criticize the system and make excuses, but you really have to step back and see if you are burning out. Not only will stress cause your practice to suffer, it is implicated in so many health issues that you may die young.

Once you establish that you are having problems dealing with stress, you have to remedy the situation. The best suggestion is to try to work toward a practice that is balanced. Don't try to treat everyone in the world. Depending upon your type of practice, consider getting a partner, or at least an associate, to allow you to take a vacation and have some time off to rejuvenate.

Health-care providers have some unique issues that can result in burnout. Some of them are difficult to identify and can lie beneath the surface resulting in generalized feelings of depression. Stress and burnout are universal and affect most everyone.

An ENT

"I just decided 'no more surgery.' The risks were too great. I didn't want to worry about losing my house to some lawsuit. Now I am happy to treat allergy and hearing problems. I work less and make out better without all of the stress."

It is important to recognize that failure is a fact of life in every health-care endeavor. Not every procedure is successful and not every patient survives. While having high ego strength helps you ignore the feelings of failure, beneath the surface it may take a toll on your psyche. It may help to have contact with fellow practitioners to share war stories and common experiences to ward off feelings of isolation and failure. Vacation time allows you to unwind and regenerate.

Maintaining a teaching affiliation and going to professional society meetings are ways for the solo practitioner to have professional contacts. Joining a group practice provides built-in professional relations that can ward off feelings of isolation and failure.

Diagnostic challenges can make you doubt your abilities, and while no one can make every diagnosis, you can take failure personally if you dwell on difficult cases. The affect on your confidence can be daunting. Fortunately, most practitioners become so busy they won't remember each failure or each diagnostic nightmare.

It should be noted that with advancing age it is not uncommon for practitioners to lose their sight or dexterity. Trying to accomplish procedures with the same level of expertise they had in earlier years may become impossible. It is extremely difficult to admit physical decline, and if practitioners don't plan for retirement, they could be forced to continue working beyond the time that they should have stopped. While still young, make sure you plan ahead so you don't have to practice when you should be enjoying the fruits of your labor.

Dealing with difficult people and staff is a strong catalyst for burnout. Learning interpersonal skills and taking courses on how to deal with difficult people may be helpful. Consider taking these courses and you will not only learn some good skills, you will be reminded that the human experience is common to all of us or there wouldn't be a need for all those courses.

Patients don't know or care what causes your coldness or rude behavior, or even that you may have cut them off while they were asking you the same question for the tenth time. They only know you aren't that doctor with the great bedside manner. If your patients know how great you usually are, they will forgive you, and because they actually feel close to you, they will often ask if something is wrong as they would a good friend. In that case you may get away with being moody on occasion. But it won't take long to use up your goodwill capital if you don't get your act together.

Doctors with good bedside manner can usually tell when they aren't themselves. If you are the oblivious type, you must learn to recognize the signs. It may be that you snap at your coworkers or employees. Perhaps a caring patient who knows this isn't you will say something. If your staff asks if something's wrong, that is a sure sign you aren't being yourself. They will often notice your bad day before you do by something as subtle as the fact that you don't say good morning.

Burnout Remedies

Vacation is a great way to unwind and regenerate. Taking several shorter vacations may provide you with more relief than waiting all year to get away for one treat. The anticipation of respite helps make the days go by faster, and the more good things you have to look forward to the better you will feel.

Consider getaway weekends if you can't schedule full weeks. Anytime away from the practice is recuperative.

Altered hours are a fabulous way to defeat the monotony of your routine. If you know that every Monday is a long hectic day, you begin to dread Monday. If surgery days are stressful, and Tuesday is surgery day... you get the idea. By having altered days and weeks, you can avoid preconceived anxiety. Consider making an A week and a B week with enough variety to keep you out of a rut.

Avoid high-stress, time-consuming, expensive hobbies. Sports, meditation, Yoga and maintaining a regular fitness program will do wonders for dealing with stress and provide you with a healthy outlet. All too often, health-care providers have so little time for themselves that they neglect their own health. Don't let high school gym be the last time you had a cardiovascular workout.

Consider avoiding dangerous hobbies and sports like motorcycling, mountain climbing, and full contact football. While some of you require intensity in your lives, the injuries from high-risk hobbies can ruin your career.

You can get much relief from stress on the racquetball, tennis, or basketball court, or by playing hockey or softball. Develop hobbies and sports skills you can continue with advancing age. You aren't going to be playing rough touch forever. A round of golf may be there for you once your knees no longer tolerate tennis. Golf can be so time consuming that it may not be right for you early on while you begin practice, but as you consider slowing down, it can offer a great getaway from the stresses of practice.

Learning some simple techniques and taking the time to relax could be the difference between an extended or shortened career. You don't have to take a formal course to learn meditation. You do have to take the time to utilize the techniques.

Yoga offers both physical and mental benefits. By taking time to relax and go into the various poses you rest your mind and the poses themselves stretch the muscles and joints to keep you flexible and fit. Like meditation, you don't have to take formal courses, but some introductory lessons would be helpful. Unless you really get into Yoga, you don't have to strive for the exotic poses that take much practice and guidance. It may be best to learn a few simple poses that help with your particular physical stresses. If you have a bad back, learn poses that stretch the back.

Besides formal Yoga postures, you can consider utilizing some basic physical therapy stretches. Anyone who has had physical therapy knows they teach many stretches that help with rehabilitation. Keep doing those that let you maintain flexibility and relieve pain.

Psychotherapy is needed when you recognize you no longer deal effectively with your stresses. While the techniques noted should keep you from getting to this point, there may come a time in your life that you need to talk with a professional. One of the biggest problems is denial or an inability to see that you need psychotherapy.

Health-care practitioners have some of the highest rates of alcohol and drug abuse, and a high suicide rate, which shows that dealing with sick people may take a toll you didn't expect when you chose this profession. Don't let yourself fall into substance abuse or succumb to untreated depression. You'd never ignore the signs in your patients and you shouldn't ignore the signs in yourself. Self-destructive behavior should not be an option.

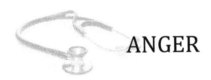

ANGER

*Doctors at a large hospital have gone on strike.
Hospital officials say they will find out what the
doctors' demands are as soon as they can get
a pharmacist to go read the picket signs!*

D octors with great bedside manner aren't supposed to be angry. Unless you are the most relaxed unflinching individual, you will get angry with patients in certain situations. Anger can affect you performance, judgment, reputation, and health. If you find yourself becoming angry too often, it may be a manifestation of burnout, and even if you have infrequent bouts of anger, you should learn to control them.

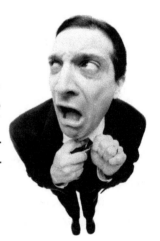

*"I called my allergist on a weekend with an emergency
concern. He called me back and didn't recognize that
I was a fellow doctor who he knew rather well. I was
shocked at his indignation that I called on the weekend.
Once he realized it was me, his demeanor changed to
that which it should be for every one of his patients
on emergency calls." Lesson: Don't act miserable just*

because you are fed up with taking after hour calls.
The person on the other end of the line is probably
pretty miserable with their emergency concerns and
fears. While these calls are often abusive and could
wait until regular office hours, you accomplish very
little by being miserable. If you really are that burned
out, hire someone to take calls for you on the weekend.

Most often, anger is directed at patients who are belligerent, ignorant, uncooperative, or inconsiderate. You have to identify what gets you upset and find remedies. The habitually late patient readily upsets the time-obsessed doctor. Because the punctuality issue is so common, the remedy is addressed in the chapter on the waiting room.

A Dental Specialist
"With difficult patients, you get mad at them,
mad at your staff and mad at yourself."

The Noncompliant Patient

Patients who don't follow directions that result in failing treatment are another major reason for resentment. You know how difficult your procedures are and how prognosis is dependent on many factors including patient compliance. While some patients are negligent and others are just not capable of following directions, you may tend to take the resultant failure as a personal affront to your ability. You can help alleviate feelings of anger and resentment by documenting each time the patient is noncompliant. Not only will it help to redirect blame when the belligerent patient wants to challenge you, it protects you from a lawsuit, and serves as a reminder that the patient may not be a good candidate for certain procedures in the future.

Fiscal Conflict

It is annoying and anger-provoking to deal with patients who incessantly complain about fees, treatment plans, and the length of therapy. By making sure there are no misunderstandings about the fees and the insurance benefits, the type of treatment and the expected number of visits, you will reduce the resentment and anger associated with this type of patient.

If a patient complains in a frequent or unreasonable way, you must have the fortitude to refuse treatment in a professional non-hostile manner. Offering a less expensive alternative treatment or suggesting that the patient seek treatment at a teaching hospital or clinic may be the best advice.

Perfectionism

Because being perfect in an imperfect world is the goal of all health-care providers, there is a particular pressure to perform at a high level of competence. Sometimes factors beyond your control make your performance suffer.

You may experience anger directed at your staff for repeated mistakes that affect your ability to deliver appropriate care. The remedy is to make sure you hire, train well, and fire as needed to develop and maintain the best staff possible. If you pay at the lower end of the pay scale you will not attract or retain the best people. Make sure you devote much energy to training your staff. Many doctors complain about incompetent staff but make no effort towards training.

A common but often unrecognized source of anger occurs when you can't perform to the level of competence required. Physical and mental decline may cause frustration and self-directed anger. It may even result in anger directed unjustifiably towards patients and staff. While physical and mental decline is usually a deficit associated with aging, it can affect practitioners at all ages if they experience any pathology that affects performance.

Something as simple as unrecognized changes in vision can affect performance. Small hand tremors, chronic back pain, stress, diminished memory, and depression are just a few of the maladies that can hurt performance and result in anger and frustration.

You must recognize physical or mental decline when it surfaces and adjust your practice accordingly. One of the best reasons to have disability insurance is to be able to leave practice when necessary rather than continue to place patients and yourself at risk.

Communication Failure

The inability of some patients to understand complex treatment plans and options, fiscal responsibilities, and general directions can be both frustrating and anger provoking for the doctor.

You have a failure to communicate when a patient asks the same question ten times. You may find yourself becoming angry. Try to smile, take a deep breath and explain again using a diagram for your records and let the patient take home a copy. Because communication is one of the major pillars of bedside manner, remedies are addressed in the chapter devoted to such issues.

Treating foreign patients presents another source of anger and frustration. There is the possible failure to communicate due the language barrier, and unfamiliar customs may be interpreted as being rude, pushy, and belligerent.

Try to be more understanding and recognize that they may have a big disadvantage in communicating. Learn a few phrases in the language of foreigners you may see often in your practice. Not only will it help make them feel more comfortable, it can disarm belligerence they may express as a result of their frustrations in communicating.

Petulance and Diminished Tolerances

Patients who have excessively low tolerance to pain or extremely high levels of anxiety can make you angry. It's often hard enough to perform technical procedures on the ideal patient, so confronting the anxious patient or the patient who jumps and screams while you are trying to concentrate can affect your performance, your emotional state, and your health.

As much as you may try to disassociate yourself from the problem patient, you must recognize you are human and entitled to have these feelings of anger and disgust. It is imperative to avoid acting on your emotions.

Because you don't see these difficult patients everyday, you don't get much practice in controlling your reaction to them. If you make a concerted effort to recognize that they are not acting difficult on purpose and that they have a true problem, you may be able to have your compassion win out. If you can't dissociate the behavior from your feelings toward the patient, you must have an escape plan in place.

The escape plan is based on a polite and courteous discussion with the patient explaining that you will not be able to treat them. You must avoid putting blame on the patient (i.e. it's not their fault that they gag, or jump or scream in the middle of a procedure), and try not to make them feel bad. This can be a touchy conversation, but as long as you know you can have it and dismiss the patient, you feel less pressured to perform under duress.

DOCTOR
"Mr. Johnson, I really would like to help you, but I'm unable to work on you when you are so jumpy. I truly understand how difficult this is for you, and I want you to get a good result, so I think it would be best to see another practitioner who has more success with anxiety (apprehension, pain control, etc.)."

DOCTOR
"Mr. Smith, I know how difficult it is for you to have this procedure done, and I truly wish that I could help you, but I'm sorry that I won't be able to do my job properly with the way you react to the needles I have to give. I think you will be able to get a much better result if

DR. ROBERT M. FLEISHER

you find a doctor who can either sedate you or give you
full anesthesia so that you can be more comfortable."

After these types of discussions, the patient will either welcome
the suggestion, offer to change his behavior, or become belligerent.
You have to be ready to deal with each scenario.

If he welcomes the suggestion, you should have the number of a
practitioner who performs the procedure under anesthesia. Do some
research into this referral since you can be held partially responsible
for making a negligent referral if the doctor malpractices.

If the patient promises to try harder, that may be all it takes to
modify their behavior to the point of becoming a reasonably decent
patient. You still have the "out" if he can't manage to perform as
required.

If the patient becomes belligerent, be apologetic and again explain in a nice, non-condescending manner that it is for his benefit.

DOCTOR
"Mr. Smith, I want you to have the best possible treatment outcome, and I can't do my job in this manner. You would have
a much better experience if you could be sedated for this
procedure, and we don't have that option in our office."

Preconceived Provocation Toward Anger

Your staff can unintentionally make you dislike your next patient
before you even meet them. They do this by telling you the negative
experience they just had in their encounter with the patient.

"Dr. Jones, Mrs. Smith refused to let me take an x-ray, and she won't
sign the informed consent or the insurance forms."

We all know how you can't wait to go in to meet Mrs. Smith. Some
of you will enter on the offense, starting the relationship on the
wrong foot. Some practitioners will instruct their assistant to go in
there and, "Tell Mrs. Smith, if she doesn't sign the forms and let you
take an x-ray, I won't see her."

That's not the solution used by the doctor with great bedside manner.

Try not to prejudice your feelings with your staff's disdain for the uncooperative patient. Sometimes the patient's inappropriate behavior is innocent and your staff may be overreacting. You should always make your own judgments and respond with the wisdom and maturity of a caring professional.

DOCTOR
"Hi, Mrs. Smith, I'm Dr. Jones. I understand
you don't want us to take an x-ray."

The patient will usually give you their reason based on the fact that they had ten other x-rays at some other office, or they may tell you about their fear of cancer. You explain the importance of why you need another x-ray and assess the degree to which this patient may be unreasonable and need to be dismissed. Once the patient meets the doctor who explains the same things the assistant told them, they usually act like a different person and acquiesce to all of the requests.

The next time your assistant tells you your new patient was rude and threw the clipboard with the patient registration form at the secretary, you will know not to be prejudiced. You will confront the patient as if he were a normal human being. If you determine that he is hostile, belligerent, threatening, uncooperative or otherwise repulsive, you should be the one to make the call about dismissing him, not your staff.

Learning that you don't have to treat everybody should take a lot of the pressure off of your psyche and help you to control your feelings. The expression of anger, frustration, resentment, and vengeance has no place in any professional relationship, and it will destroy any semblance of bedside manner. It is much better to dismiss the patient who riles you than to punish them by childish, vindictive acts such as making them wait longer to see you or treating them inappropriately.

NAME RECOGNITION

A resident approached an elderly man
on a gurney in the E.R.
Resident: "Do you know who I am?"
Old Guy: "Sure, you're the doctor,
but I don't know your name."
Resident: "So what brought you to the E.R.?"
Old Guy: "An ambulance."

Branding is the commercial concept of developing a recognizable reputation that is marketable and has value in terms of **goodwill**. Professional practice incorporates the same concepts. Doctors, hospitals, and clinics all value their reputation, and branding offers increased patient flow, research grants, and overall fiscal valuation of the entity. Most private practitioners are more concerned with their professional reputation out of pride and often don't think of the business benefits derived from such branding that comes from their good reputation. There is nothing more potent for increasing the reputation and branding of the health-care professional than having a great bedside manner.

"I never would have expected to see the day that patients had no clue as to who their doctor is. They could care less nowadays. All they worry about is the ten-

dollar co-payment. When I started out, they would
only see the doctor they had grown to love and respect.
They knew my name."
The lament of an older doctor.

————————————

For the provider in solo practice there is only one name on the door, making name recognition easy. In today's professional practice, you may be the new associate or one of many practitioners in a group practice. To remain anonymous in a large practice will not serve you well. You need to create name recognition for yourself. If your compensation is based on productivity, it makes good economic sense to have patients requesting to see you and only you. If you decide to go on your own and you are not encumbered by a restrictive covenant, your patients will follow.

In a practice with more than one provider, you must make every effort to make sure the patient knows your name. You must be subtle and not get carried away in flaunting your name or you run the risk of looking egotistical. It's easy to have your name mentioned and if you provide appropriate scripting it will get your name out there along with your reputation of having a great bedside manner.

The first opportunity to mention your own name is upon initial introduction, but it is often missed or forgotten by the already apprehensive patient. Another opportunity presents when using humor that gets your patient to laugh as described in the comedy chapter. After they laugh at any of your comical lines, it's easy to say, "Just make sure you don't tell your friends you were laughing during root canal treatment with Dr. Fleisher, or we'll both get in trouble." Not only does this get your name repeated in case they forgot the ten other times your staff mentioned it, but it also gets another laugh.

Besides mentioning your own name, you must make sure your staff mentions your name on all appropriate occasions. This begins with the very first contact by phone. "Mr. Smith, your appointment will be with doctor Fleisher, on Thursday, July 11." When the patient arrives, your receptionist should repeat your name, "Good morning,

Mr. Smith. You'll be seeing Dr. Fleisher this morning. We'll be with you shortly."

"The doctor will be with you shortly. You can have a seat and fill out these forms," is the greeting most often used and it is totally inappropriate.

When your patient is brought back to the treatment room, your assistant should again mention your name before and after they have done their preliminary workup. "Good morning. Mr. Smith. I see you're here to see Dr. Fleisher." They take the medical history or get an x-ray, and when they are ready to leave the room they say, "Dr. Fleisher will be with you shortly."

There should be no reason for a patient to ask, "Which doctor are you?" If they do, your staff is not doing their job, the patient didn't hear the staff's numerous attempts to mention your name, or the patient just wants to be sure whom they are seeing.

When they do ask, "Which doctor are you?" reply with, "I'm not a witch doctor, I think you may have the wrong office." Not only will they soon know your name, they know you have a sense of humor and it sets the stage for the fast bonding that humor engenders.

If the patient needs another appointment, make sure your receptionist again mentions your name. "Here's your appointment card. Dr. Fleisher will look forward to seeing you on the twenty-sixth."

Some people just can't remember names–especially if you are in a specialty practice, where the patients don't see you often. Even if the patient can't remember your name, they may remember a particular trait that keeps them seeking you and only you. Always be distinctive.

Name recognition is what makes up the nebulous concept of goodwill. It is often goodwill that is bought and sold when professional practices change hands. Make sure you have an identifiable name, as it adds value to your goodwill.

Many modern healthcare facilities utilize a **practice or facility name** and intentionally avoid the names of the doctors in any marketing. This serves the purpose of allowing for a constant turnover of practitioners, and it keeps the "goodwill" value in the hands of the corporate owner i.e. a hospital or usually a large practice that wants to avoid personality preferences by the patients. It is much easier to sell a practice once a doctor relocates or dies if the practice has a well known corporate name. This bodes poorly for the individual practitioner who wants to build a name recognition practice. And while it may be fine for institutions, it also bodes poorly for healthcare where the personal touch is lost to the persona of big business.

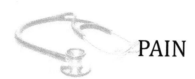 PAIN

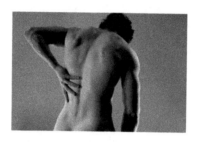

A woman goes to her doctor who verifies that she is pregnant. This is her first pregnancy. The doctor asks her if she has any questions. She replies, "Well, I'm a little worried about the pain.
How much will childbirth hurt?"
The doctor answered, "Well, that varies from woman to woman and pregnancy to pregnancy and besides, it's difficult to describe pain."
"I know, but can't you give me some idea?" she asks.
"Grab your upper lip and pull it out a little..."
"Like this?"
"A little more..."
"Like this?"
"No. A little more..."
"Like this?"
"Yes. Does that hurt?"
"A little bit."
"Now stretch it over your head!"

If the procedures you perform are known to involve pain, you have a built-in bedside manner generator. Just perform pain-free procedures. Patients rave about many practitioners who have absolutely no bedside manner, as defined throughout this book, just because they don't hurt them during a procedure perceived to be painful.

The dentist and most dental specialties have this advantage. Since dentistry is probably the most feared health-care need, patients who survive without any pain will go back over and over, even if the doctor has no personality or people skills.

While performing pain-free procedures offers a way to be loved without all the usual skill sets, it also presents many challenges. There are reasons people fear dentistry. It does, at times, hurt. Everything from administering an injection to working on a tooth that can't be numbed puts tremendous pressure on the dentist and justifies the anxiety and fears the patient experiences.

The importance of learning techniques to give virtually painless, highly effective injections is the key to winning over the patient. Leaning advanced techniques of sedation or general anesthesia, when indicated, should be considered since some cases involve unavoidable pain with conventional pain control modalities.

The dentist isn't the only one delivering potentially painful procedures. Many other areas of practice are not as feared, so unsuspecting patients end up being catheterized, scoped, or otherwise probed and prodded painfully, but without the preconceived fear associated with going to the dentist.

Whatever services you perform, learn to do them as painlessly as possible, and you will have a patient for life. Make sure you utilize the latest and greatest techniques for pain control. Give extra anesthesia and wait longer for it to take effect if necessary. Don't rush when it comes to pain control. When you think the procedure can't be done without pain, or if you believe the psyche of the patient is such that he is not a good candidate for the procedure, consider referring him to someone who can provide sedation if you don't utilize that modality.

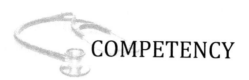# COMPETENCY

---

*Psychiatrist to nurse: "Just say we're very
busy, don't keep saying, 'It's a madhouse.'"*

While in the beginning, competency was not defined as a critical component of bedside manner; it is the essence of being a truly great provider. Everyone in the health-care industry should strive to be the most competent provider around.

Creed of Competency: *It is the duty of all health-care providers to be the best that they can be, to limit practice to areas of expertise and competency, and to seek quality continuing education to make sure that they remain at the leading edge of the science and art of practice. It is the obligation of every practitioner to know when to refer patients for specialty care.*

Competency should be a matter of fact in all endeavors. When you fly, you expect the pilot and crew to be highly competent. Patients expect the same from their doctors. The duty of the examining and licensing boards is to make sure doctors are competent and remain competent throughout their years of practice. Unfortunately, competency is not always guaranteed. While states have made a good attempt at maintaining competency by requiring continuing education, very little is done to police the profession. As a result, there are incompetent practitioners.

Even with the lack of guaranteed competency that we know exists, the public still maintains the belief that doctors are competent. Ironically, every patient likes to believe that not only are their doctors competent, but they are the best. Fortunately, most times they are at least correct on the former assumption.

I have known several incompetent practitioners cherished by their patients. I have seen waiting rooms filled to capacity with wait times of, literally, hours. If you told the patients that there's a doctor next door who could see them immediately, not one of them would leave. What these doctors lacked in competency they made up in bedside manner. That's loyalty! But that is not the type of practitioner you want to be.

CONCLUSION

The doctor tells the patient he has a bad heart. The fellow says, "I want another opinion." The doctor says, "Okay, you're ugly too."

Bedside manner is an amalgamation of many factors. It is not just a great personality, a talent for humor, or an abundance of compassion. It is all those qualities and many more. It can be learned and practiced to make each and every health-care provider more likeable and successful. Just being a good healer is not enough. Bedside manner addresses the psychological aspects of patient care. In a fast-paced, impersonal world, the psyche needs healing just as much as the body.

By recognizing the importance of being a complete practitioner, you will make it a point to learn the techniques described. Take the time to become aware of all your patients' needs, and what they require and seek from the doctor-patient relationship.

Everyone should make an effort to sharpen their interpersonal skills as much as they should stay at the forefront of their field of patient care. Both qualities make the best doctors.

Dr. FLEISHER was born in Arlington, Virginia and grew up in Philadelphia, Pennsylvania. After receiving his Bachelor of Arts in psychology and his D.M.D. at Temple University, Dr. Fleisher attended the University of Pennsylvania where he received his specialty training in endodontics. Dr. Fleisher has taught at Temple University, the University of Pennsylvania, and currently teaches at the Albert Einstein Medical Center in Philadelphia. After twenty-five years of teaching his winning formulas to many generations of practitioners at this hospital-based endodontic program, Dr. Fleisher was inducted into the Maimonides Society.

Dr. Fleisher maintained a full-time private practice for over thirty years. It had grown to become the largest endodontic practice in the state. Treating over thirty thousand patients, Dr. Fleisher has had the unique opportunity to interact with patients who, for the most part, were not happy to see him. After a few minutes that attitude changed, and pretty soon, Dr. Fleisher had his patients laughing during the course of root canal therapy. He boasts that while all famous comedians can make people laugh, he too can make people laugh, but none of them can do root canal therapy.

By developing and instituting practice management systems that go beyond the typical financial instructions and ways to get more patients, Dr. Fleisher teaches office design, employee and doctor scripts, interpersonal techniques, and compassion to build a practice and to make sure patients remain loyal, are kept happy, and love you.

For More Information and To Add Your

Comments, Ideas and Suggestions About

Bedside Manner

visit

www.bedsidemanner.info

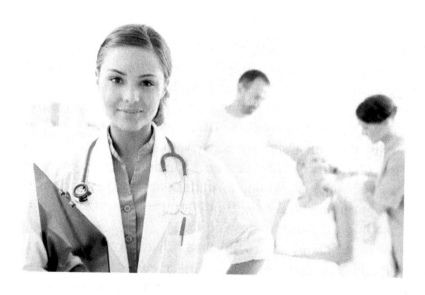

Also by Dr. Robert Fleisher

Forty Something
A Guide through Mid-Life and Mid-Life Crisis

Fifty Something
You Still Have Time to Redeem Your Body and Soul from Past Neglect

visit

www.mid-lifecrisis.com

Printed in the USA
CPSIA information can be obtained
at www.ICGtesting.com
LVHW020553201223
766796LV00003B/173